FOOD SMART!
Eat Your Way to Better Health

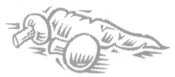

CHERYL TOWNSLEY

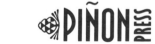

P.O. Box 35007, Colorado Springs, Colorado 80935

Library of Congress Catalog Card Number:
    94-25604
ISBN 08910-98399

Cover and interior illustrations: Amy Bryant

Some of the anecdotal illustrations in this book are true to
life and are included with the permission of the persons
involved. All other illustrations are composites of real situations, and any resemblance to people living or dead is
coincidental.

This publication is designed to provide accurate and
authoritative information in regard to the subject matter
covered. It is sold with the understanding that the author
and the publisher are not engaged in rendering legal,
accounting, or other professional service. If legal advice or
other expert assistance is required, the services of a com-
petent professional person should be sought. *From a
Declaration of Principles jointly adopted by a Committee
of the American Bar Association and a Committee of
Publishers.*

Townsley, Cheryl.
        Food smart! : eat your way to better health /
    Cheryl Townsley
        p.   cm.
        Includes bibliographical references.
        ISBN 0-89109-839-9
        1. Nutrition. 2. Health. I. Title.
    RA784.T685   1994
    613.2—dc20   94-25604
                                                CIP

Printed in the United States of America

2 3 4 5 6 7 8 9 10 11 12 13 14 15/99 98 97 96 95 94

Contents

To parents who blessed me with life,
To a brother who is more than a brother,
To a dear husband who is my very best friend,
To a precious little girl who is a blessing to us all,
To my God who gave me life and gave it back again renewed,
I dedicate this book with love.

May you each be blessed as you have so richly blessed me.
I love you dearly.

Acknowledgments

"Mom, you're *always* on the computer," was an often-heard complaint from my daughter, Anna. How thrilled my family is to have me finished with this set of writing deadlines. Anna, our special little girl, and Forest, my dear, supportive husband, have helped balance the home front during my computer marathon days. Thanks for being the best family a woman could ever ask for.

Thanks to Dr. Peter Petropulos for working with our family to save my life. Without your expertise, patience, and support, I would probably not be alive to share my story.

To my other health-team players—Mary Hageman, Ellen Meyers-Martin, Dr. George Juetersonke, Dr. Wolfe, Lynda Rodenbaugh—may I say thanks for helping me move further in the process of restoring my health. Your individual attention, compassion, and training have enriched me forever.

Thanks to one great publishing staff for all of their tireless efforts from editing to marketing. A better team of qualified professionals and dedicated individuals would be hard to find. A special thanks to Traci Mullins for her commitment to excellence.

To friends and family members too numerous to mention, I offer you a public acknowledgment of my thanks and my personal prayers. May you be richly blessed for all that you have invested in my life.

Introduction

The doctor of the future will give no medicine, but will interest his patients in the care of the human frame, in diet, and in the cause and prevention of disease.

Thomas A. Edison

When I awoke in the hospital bed with my family around me, I slowly remembered what had happened. Yes, I had tried to kill myself. My mind had become my enemy instead of my long-time friend. My emotions were totally unreliable and had basically shut down. My overweight, tired, sick body just didn't care, or have the energy to care, about anything. The bottle of pills seemed the only solution. But, even that I had failed to do correctly, or so I thought.

To leave the hospital under those conditions required that I see a psychiatrist. As he recommended medication to help me deal with my mood swings, I foggily knew there had to be another way. Pills had gotten me into the hospital. I didn't want more pills; I wanted help identifying and solving my problems.

Dear friends referred me to a nutritionist. Should I talk to

9

him? What did I have to lose? He would probably be like everyone else, but I could at least try. As the nutritionist competently answered each and every one of my questions, I began to have hope in spite of my best intentions to stay uninterested.

Now, years later, I am reaping more and more of the fruit of that first step. The process has taken time, effort, and commitment. But, oh, the joy of feeling good and being able to think! I would never choose to go back to my old ways.

This book is my opportunity to share my story with you. My prayer is that you will never have to go through what I went through. And, if you are where I was, I want you to know that there is hope and there are options. Becoming healthier is a possibility for any person reading this book.

Since that day, I have become healthier. I have been able to share what I have learned through my books: *Lifestyle for Health*, *Meals in 30 Minutes*, and *Kid's Favorites*. Our bimonthly *Lifestyle for Health Newsletter* helps people develop their understanding of health and nutrition, while getting new recipes and a little dose of humor. If you would like to contact me, please do so at:

Cheryl Townsley
Lifestyle for Health
P.O. Box 3871
Littleton, CO 80161-3871
(303)771-9357

Although I am not a doctor, I would like to interest you in a little prevention, or maybe solve the mystery of why you don't feel so good today. So, let's get a cup of tea, sit back, and talk like friends. I have an interesting story I think you will enjoy.

Part One
The Quest for Health

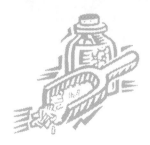

CHAPTER ONE

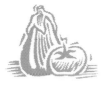

So Ugly!

I looked in the mirror and said aloud, "Cheryl, you are so ugly! God, I just can't live like this anymore." I proceeded to take a handful of sleeping pills, one at a time. I lay down on the bed. From somewhere deep within, I summoned the clearness of mind to remember Forest's phone number. I dialed the number, told his secretary to send him home, and then passed out.

What had happened to my life? What had gone wrong? Let's take a look at my life just a few years before.

WHERE HAD IT STARTED?

Graduating from high school with honors, I seemed to be able to do anything I set my mind to. College seemed the natural step to take in my pursuit of success. The first in my immediate family to finish high school and college, I felt a strong desire to succeed in these new, unknown waters.

In college, I took eighteen to twenty-seven hours a semester when the normal load was twelve to fifteen. I added ten to thirty hours of outside work a week to my study and class load. The foundation of the fast-track life was being well laid.

Graduating in three and a half years with honors and as a Phi Beta Kappa (National Honor Society) member seemed to be a good way to start my professional career.

With great self-discipline I jumped into teaching junior high home economics. I began to learn that working at a job that didn't match my interests could be very stressful. I loved home ec, but I couldn't understand why I didn't like to teach it. I would be physically ill on Friday night just thinking about the fact that I had to go back to my classroom on Monday morning. This didn't make for very many exciting weekends!

After a year, I decided to try my hand at dress design and custom tailoring. As that enterprise began to grow, I realized that I had never learned much about how to run a business. Being performance-oriented, I decided to continue to build my business while also getting additional education in business operations. I headed back to college to earn a double degree in computer science and business management.

After obtaining these degrees, I began my "business career" in the corporate world. Over the next several years I climbed the corporate ladder with various corporations. I found myself winning numerous awards in the technical arena and later in the sales arena.

Sales seemed to be the perfect match to my skills and interests. Even in my twenties my personal belief in a product gave me the conviction to make sales presentations to any person, regardless of job title or age. What a thrill when a vice president of a Fortune 500 company would decide to sign a new contract with me.

Earning in excess of $70,000 by the age of twenty-nine, I felt I had the world by the horns. I was flying throughout the country as a national product manager for a computer services company. My personal and business schedule began to merge into one hectic "day." I would have dry cleaning to pick up in one city and personal mail being sent to another, as I scheduled executive presentations and local sales meetings in a third city. I had a house sitter who would stock the refrigerator for my return home, as well as pick me up from and return me to the airport. Success, money, travel—it all seemed great.

PROFESSIONAL SUCCESS, PERSONAL FAILURE

A small problem had arisen during this time. I had divorced—twice. Somehow, I felt that my professional success would eventually help me deal with the shambles in my personal life. Certainly a little stress in my twenties and thirties was worth the price of "success."

I moved on to start my own consulting company. I completed several contracts, but the stress of satisfying those clients was growing. During this time I met, dated, and subsequently married my husband, Forest. Within five months I was pregnant. That was not part of my business plan, to say the least.

Stress began to mount as my pregnancy limited me to my bed for seven months. Unemployed, Forest was selling off antiques, a car, and other paraphernalia to buy groceries. The pregnancy was the beginning of the decline in my physical health. Or, I should say, it was the first time I noticed or could "see" my health decline.

Our daughter was born in 1984, a month early. She was healthy and beautiful, and an easy baby. My nerves could never have tolerated a fussy baby.

After she turned five months, I worked for one year. During that time of consulting assignments, my stress load increased. My weight began increasing and our finances deteriorated further.

Following that, various circumstances required that I stay home and be a full-time mother. The major problem with that decision was all of my identity had been in my career and professional success. Who was I, if I wasn't working?

I tried to start a computer company, in which I failed miserably. I disappointed investors, coworkers, and myself. I could no longer achieve a goal just because I had set it. Facing that stark reality seemed insurmountable. I was no longer able to mask emotions and fears with grim self-determination.

One day I was waiting for Forest at his office. He was out making sales calls, which was his job. I could not figure out how to get home, a mile and a half away. I was furious with Forest by the time he came back to the office. He had not known I was there waiting for him. I could not stem my anger at being left alone. I was afraid. I had traversed New York's subway system, Europe, and many other places. Now I could not find my way home in suburban Denver. What was happening to me?

Having returned from Forest's office on another day, the scene in front of the mirror occurred. Suicide seemed the only way to deal with career disappointments, growing financial problems, deteriorating health, and my identity crisis. What I had always believed and done just didn't seem to work anymore. Yet to not believe or do what I believed was unthinkable. I cried out in front of the mirror; I just let go. The reflection of "ugliness" was too much. I could no longer deal with my life and the mess I had made of it. I slowly, hopelessly swallowed the pills.

As they treated me in the hospital, I remember overhearing bits and pieces of the conversation. The nurse had me drink liquid charcoal to coat my stomach from the effect of the pills. As I dutifully drank it she commented to Forest in amazement: "She is drinking all of it! No one ever drinks it so well or so quickly."

Forest responded, "She always does it just right." What a prophetic and insightful statement. So true and yet so sad.

THE PROBLEMS GROW

My health continued to decline. I became emotionally depressed and mentally muddled. Forest would make me promise each morning that I would be there when he came home that night. He knew that if I gave my word I would keep it and not try another suicide attempt . . . at least that day.

I was eating less and gaining weight. I contemplated looking for a job to help with our finances. But we never knew if I would have a "good" day and actually perform long enough to get through an entire interview. Besides, my career clothes weren't fitting and we had no money to outfit me anew. My professional image was becoming pretty shabby, to say the least.

Emotionally I was out of balance. I would cry over everything. This woman who in the past had coolly and calmly presented multimillion-dollar computer proposals to vice presidents could not handle a phone call. A call from a bill collector would cause me to shut down emotionally and physically for days. No longer did my award-winning self-discipline seem to be enough to hold me together.

Besides my weight, emotional, and mental problems, my skin was breaking out all over my body. It would itch, and I would scratch until my skin bled. What little beauty I thought I might have had seemed to have totally evaporated.

Whatever I ate seemed to bloat or constipate me. I craved sweets and bread, yet nothing satisfied or tasted good once I put it in my mouth.

What could I do? We tried everything we knew. We tried doctor after doctor. They told us there was nothing medically wrong. Nothing medically wrong? Why couldn't I function? I used to be a functional, intelligent, alert, stable woman. What had gone wrong? Had I only imagined my life before this time? My life seemed totally out of control and hopeless. What a scary place to be.

To add to this stress, we had gone through bankruptcy. We also went through foreclosure on a house that I had bought prior to our marriage. By this time we had closed Forest's business and he was now unemployed. We were living on $850 month ... a far cry from my over $70,000-a-year income just a few years before.

Where could we turn? All of the doors seemed to be shut.

As I looked back over my journal for this time period, an entry for October 6, 1988, stands out. I had written,

> I feel numb; there seems to be no feeling or desires left in me. There are no tears, no anger, only tiredness. No desires, no dreams ... nothing seems to matter. Whether I clean the house today, tomorrow, or next week, it doesn't seem to matter. We do have a meal every day and clean dishes. Every now and then I sew. There's no rush, just a few things to do before Christmas. My hands are breaking

out again. I have no idea what to do anymore.

Everything I have done this past year created disaster. I am right back to where I was last October, three Octobers ago, four Octobers ago. The same problems, only now they are more severe. In addition, my health has deteriorated. What does God want from me now? I don't even feel lost anymore. You have to be going somewhere to get lost. . . . I no longer know what "my lot" or "my work" in life is. Any life in me, beyond mere physical existence, must be given to me . . . I can't do it anymore.

You may not identify with the hopelessness I felt—physically, mentally, or emotionally. Perhaps you just don't feel as well as you think you could. Or maybe you're concerned about how diet and lifestyle may affect your health down the road. Perhaps you're plagued with a level of fatigue that is starting to concern you. Maybe regular depression or a sense of hopelessness vexes you. Maybe a roller coaster ride of weight gain and weight loss is discouraging you.

Regardless of your current situation, the keys to health that I have discovered can work for you. You don't have to wait for a crisis to begin unlocking your health. Improved health is a joyful process that no one should miss out on.

GOOD NEWS!

A good friend of ours mentioned a nutritionist to us. We decided we had nothing to lose, so I made an appointment with him. I asked Forest to go with me. I had become so disillusioned with "experts" that my manner with them bordered on rude and obnoxious. I went, armed with my questions and my hostility.

The nutritionist calmly answered each and every question related to my physical problems. He treated me like an intelligent person capable of understanding these problems. He said he could help. He informed us of the probable roots for the physical symptoms, what needed to be done, and how it could be approached.

What were his comments? He told us that my body was highly toxic (poisoned on the inside), my immune system was broken, and my digestive system lacked the necessary digestive enzymes. Much of this made no sense to me at the time. It basically came down to the fact that I was very sick.

He suggested taking time to cleanse my body of its toxicity. He also said I would go through a building-up process to strengthen the various systems in my body. Nutritious meals would be critical to building my overall health. He estimated that it would take six to twelve months to achieve these two goals.

Now, wait a minute, I thought. He was talking to a former home ec teacher. I knew about nutrition (or so I thought). Why, I had learned about it in school. Besides, I had been changing my poor eating habits from my old corporate days. By the time we saw our nutritionist, I thought I was cooking extremely "healthy" meals. We were eating a few vegetables, cutting down on fat, and using whole-wheat flour. What more could there be to "health food" and nutritious meals? Surely our current diet paralleled good nutrition.

He continued talking. Foreign concepts like cleansing, fasting, supplements, herbs, and toxins were presented. Was he just strange, or did he have some real wisdom? How would it feel to be physically clean and healthy? Would that help my mental faculties? What about my roller coaster emotions? Would I ever be able to perform in a career again? It was all so new and different. I had no idea what was ahead for me.

Our nutritionist made the comment to us that we are today what we have been eating for years. We reap what we sow.

What had I sown over the first thirty years of my life? As I looked back, I saw a pattern. Achievement and performance were everything to me. I would work inhumane hours if it meant I would meet my goal or schedule.

Did it matter if I reached the goal and died in the process? As I looked back on my college schedule, I could see little merit in my accomplishments when weighed against the ulcer conditions that they caused. What if I had waited one more semester to graduate (graduating in the "normal" four years instead of three and a half)? Maybe I would have realized that junior high teaching was not for me, and I could have avoided a year and a half of additional stress.

I had always seen myself as a basically healthy, energetic person. When I became chronically ill, I had no coping skills. Looking back on my fast-paced corporate life, I can see that I ate whatever looked good on the high-end restaurant menu. Although I loved to cook, time never permitted such a luxury. With money not an issue, I ate most of my meals out. I never thought of the fat, sugar, or cholesterol count. My weight was fairly constant. I felt good, so what difference did it make what I ate?

If my schedule dictated that I be out late and up early to catch the next plane, I did it. If I had to be in meetings all day and couldn't exercise, so be it.

In other areas of my life I had learned that *what you deposit is directly related to what is available for withdrawal.* I understood this principle in the realm of banking (my checkbook and savings accounts), but I had no comprehension of it in regard to health or other less tangible areas of my life.

LET'S GO FOR IT!

Could we actually do what the nutritionist was suggesting? Could we afford to do it on $850 a month? What if it didn't work? So many questions raced (or maybe crawled) through my foggy mind. Yet, what if he really could help and I could get better? Was it worth the effort? Was it worth the potential disappointment if it didn't work? What about the cost to our already depleted budget?

The crisis I was in dictated our response to those questions. What did I have to lose? With little consideration, we decided to plunge ahead full force with this "nutritional approach." In one day, we made the decision to change our diet. We moved quickly to transition our pantry from our "old" food to the newly allowed foods. We were motivated by my life-and-death situation. Within a few weeks we began to see significant changes. Within six months I had lost most of my excess weight, my skin had cleared, my emotions had begun to stabilize, and I had begun making decisions. These changes felt enormous compared to where I had been.

Forest joined me in our nutritional program. We found that he was actually physically sicker than I was. When we questioned our nutritionist, he made an interesting comment. He said that women, due to their monthly hormone changes, will manifest their physical and emotional problems sooner. Men will wait and keel over with a heart attack.

We found that Forest's asthmatic problems were actually far more advanced than we thought. Following our time of cleansing and diet changes, Forest also dropped weight, came off his asthma medication (which he had been taking for over thirty years), and had a much more youthful appearance.

As I made nutritional changes, I also began to reflect on my mental and emotional status. Some of my mental and emotional "opportunities to change" came because of the radical change in our physical diet. When I was having a stressful day, a bag of chocolate-chip cookies was no longer an option. (How unfair!) When I felt angry at Forest or depressed with our finances (we were still on a very tight budget), I could no longer go out to eat a big pizza. (Such deprivation!) My commitment to our new nutritional plan forced me to begin to look at my responses to mental and emotional pressures. I began to go beyond what seemed "fair" and "normal." I started being honest with myself, as best I could.

One advantage of being unemployed is that you have time. I had time to begin to explore why I was behaving the way I was. I began to explore my feelings. I found that many of my mind-sets and emotional reactions were merely habits. The good news about habits is that they can be changed. The bad news is that changing habits takes time. I began to develop and apply the principles that I will share with you in this book. These healing principles applied to my mental and emotional healing as well as my physical healing.

I began to allow myself the freedom to do less. The house did not have to be perfect. I learned to have a few piles lying around. That may seem like a small deal, but it wasn't for me. I had been a person who made sure the vacuum lines in our white carpet were perfectly even each time I vacuumed. I learned to set more reasonable goals and forgive myself if I decided not to pursue them.

When I was tempted to explode or isolate myself emotionally, I took time and dealt with the issue. In the past, I usually suppressed my emotions. Since most emotions were "bad," I had to learn how to acknowledge them without becoming a slave to them. Both the mental and emotional healing took time.

As I worked at getting healthier, people began to comment on my progress. I looked better. Equally important, people began to notice and acknowledge that I seemed like a more mellow, peaceful person. What a compliment to a former type-A, driver, choleric, performance-obsessed professional! The effort was paying off. I still have drive and ambition, but I am learning how to balance them with compassion and relationship. I am making healthier food choices while balancing those choices with life in a real world that is not always perfect. Each step is progress. I am learning to enjoy the process and not just anxiously await the goal.

I am continually sharing that process with others. As I work with individuals and families, I usually recommend that they take as long as a year, or even longer, to make this kind of transition. A person or family not in a crisis situation has the luxury of taking more time. Most of all, I encourage these people to determine *why* they want to change their lifestyle and food choices. As they explore their real motivation to change, they begin to develop the internal desire to begin making changes here and there. Before they know it, they have changed several things and are actually seeing enough fruit from their efforts to warrant continuing on in the adventure.

SHARING THE GOOD NEWS

We have always enjoyed having people over to eat in our home, so I became challenged to take our "health food" and make it palatable for our junk-food friends. What good is health food if it looks strange and tastes lousy? The "Townsley Cafe" became, and still is, a favorite place to eat for many people.

People around us began to notice the changes in us. They began to ask us what had happened. They wanted to know what we were doing differently. Our story began to circulate. We began to share the process we had followed to recapture our health.

These friends would begin to share their experiences. Over and over I would hear how they had tried "diet programs" or eating healthier or this and that—only to fail, one more time. I could understand their sense of hopelessness. I had been there, too.

As I got healthier, I began to teach in a local health-food store. Even learning how to do a part-time (one-day-a-month) job was a process for me. When I went in for the interview, I took a business plan of ideas with me, in addition to my résumé. The cooking-school administrator later told me of her reactions. She showed my "package" to her boss and wondered why I was applying for a once-a-month instructor position. I was still learning to just be me and not have the need to show every credential in order to gain acceptance.

While I was teaching these classes, the students began to ask for copies of my recipes. Friends requested recipes and advice on making changes in their food choices. So, I began to write and publish cookbooks on health food that actually tasted good. In the past I had feverishly pursued professional success so that I could accrue fame and wealth. I determined with this new business in the health-food industry to do it differently. It took lots of falling down and getting up to begin to learn how to run a business and still maintain balance in my health and with my family.

I began to allow myself the freedom to fail so that I could learn to walk in new principles of health. Having always resisted any form of failure, I had locked myself out of many opportunities to grow and improve. As I grew in my health, many people asked me to share how I had done it. As I shared my experiences with others, I began to notice similarities between their stories and mine. The gaping holes in our attempts to become healthy began to take shape into consistent patterns. The keys that I found working for me appeared to fit these gaping holes. Time after time I have watched these principles meet the needs of individuals and families desiring to make health changes successfully.

Many of the people I work with have read numerous books or articles on health. Most of these books tend to be of the crisis or doom-and-gloom variety. If they do not lean toward this negative approach, they are often filled with a huge amount of complicated, overwhelming information. Most people respond to this information in one of three ways.

The first is with *rebellion*. Their first response is, "You aren't going to tell me what I can and can't eat. I have a *right* to eat whatever I want to eat! And furthermore, I *will* eat what I want to eat." These people dismiss the whole package of health as irrelevant, unnecessary, and unimportant. Their resolve grows with each new article or book. I have found that as I share my story, without judgment or pressure, their interest is piqued. As I share the information contained in part 2 of this book, they begin to contemplate their own situation. Over time, if they are given the freedom to quietly consider this approach, they begin to open.

A second way people respond is with *fear.* They hear the gloomy forecast and the crisis health story and they immediately fear for their lives. The one immediate result of fear is paralysis. These people quickly become overwhelmed and paralyzed in their fear. They may overreact and try to do everything at once. When that fails, which it does, their fear begins to mushroom. They become obsessed with every symptom, every possibility, and every expert opinion. I have found that it helps to take these folks by the hand and help them identify *one* place to start. I constantly remind them that this is a process of many steps and it takes time. It is okay to take time. Each step is an improvement from where they have been. Encouragement is a critical piece of their progress. Part 2 of this book will help you understand how essential balance and encouragement are.

The third way people respond is with *excitement*. How many times have *you* gotten excited about a speaker or author; gone out and purchased every book, tool, or resource that he or she recommended; and then, in a few days, weeks, or months, found yourself right back where you started? As I see this tendency in people, I remind them that health is a process, not a destination. Health is not instant; it will take time. Health results from lifestyle changes, not from an immediate dose of anything.

I have worked with people responding in each of these ways and have been amazed at the results. The principles that worked for me began to work for them. As people started implementing these principles, I began to notice significant, and more importantly, *lasting changes in their health.*

Now it's time to share some of those key principles with you. May they help the multitude of Americans who are:

▶ tired of the swings in weight gain and weight loss
▶ suffering from depression, mood swings, and a sense of hopelessness
▶ tired of repeated failures in their attempts to improve their health
▶ unsure where or how to start changing their diet
▶ sick with chronic degenerative diseases
▶ unsuccessfully trying to get a spouse or family member to change his or her approach to health
▶ tired of living a life of constant stress and don't know how to get off the merry-go-round
▶ suffering from chronic fatigue
▶ on a tight money and time budget and still want to eat healthfully
▶ interested in their health options

You can be successful in your process of becoming healthy. I am proof that, no matter how far you sink, there is a way out. Best of all, if you aren't in a crisis, you have the opportunity to reap the benefits more quickly. As I share my healing experiences and the key principles that helped me unlock my health process, I trust that you, too, will become healthier. These principles have worked for our family and numerous others. We share them with you as a typical American family, not as a medical or professional health-care provider.

As you begin to consider changing parts of your lifestyle, you will be confronted with many subtle aspects of our cultural conditioning. Most of us are unaware of that conditioning and its influence in our daily decisions. We are conditioned to believe that busy-ness is a sign of success and being in high demand. We take pride in working hard—fifty to sixty-plus hours a week—to earn a better living for ourselves. We push ourselves in every area of life to get more—more time, more money, more success, more status, and on and on. But we also get more stress and all of its consequences.

We work hard, but we often fail to work smart. Failing to work smart, we reap a lifetime of stressful existence. We miss out on the daily satisfaction and fulfillment of living. For example, our culture encourages us to eat fast meals to save time. We save so much time that we die earlier. We are told we deserve a break today, so we "veg" out in front of television. We "veg" out so long that we forget how to communicate with others. We are told to work hard at our jobs so that we can be promoted to better jobs. We work so hard that when we blink, our life has disappeared, our children have grown, and we are not much farther than when we started.

Becoming healthier has brought me much-needed revelation on this cultural conditioning. Over time we begin to accept our culture's conditions as normal. We think everybody else is doing it, so we should, too. No longer do I blindly accept this system without questioning and thinking. I have stopped and taken time to become aware of my own beliefs. In the process, I have begun to redefine what is acceptable and normal for me. As a result, I have accepted the responsibility for my own health and my own life. I am no longer a victim.

In the past I used my mind to push myself into aggressive self-development programs. I was constantly thinking ahead. I did as many things at one time as possible (and sometimes even impossible) in order to be efficient. I developed the question-able ability to split my focus in many directions. This produced a form of double-mindedness, which, in concert with the constant mental pressure to perform, brought confusion and eventually my mental breakdown.

Today, I take time to do one thing at a time. I have learned to relax and think through what needs to be done. Thinking through my options, instead of just reacting and pushing, has caused my thinking to be more clear. I am able to evaluate the short- and long-term consequences of decisions before having to experience those consequences. When I see mental pressure and double-mindedness raise their ugly heads, I realize that I am slipping into old habits. Just taking the time to recognize that encourages me to slow down and refocus on what is really important.

In the past I guarded my emotions to prevent hurt. Becoming self-sufficient seemed a worthy goal for my ultimate success. I pushed myself to achieve in every area of my life so that I could be accepted by . . . somebody. This direction brought divorce, alienation, emptiness, and aloneness. As the proverbial saying goes, "I had the world's success and no one to share it with."

Today, I am learning to be myself. I'm finding that Cheryl really is a nice person. I am learning how to take time for other people and how to be a friend. I am learning that a family can be a team that is stronger than its individual components. The health-ier I get, the more I experience an entirely new realm of rela-tionship and acceptance.

In the past I expected a doctor or other professional to fix my health. I felt that I had the right to eat whatever I wanted, whenever I wanted. After all, I was a busy person. I wanted instant results, pills for headaches, quick fixes for weight prob-lems, and miracle cures for my depression. I am now learning to be responsible for my own health symptoms. I am learning to make smart food choices that nourish and build my body. As a result I have more stamina and much less downtime. I now look forward to each day.

As I get healthier and less bound to this cultural system of pressure and stress, I am finding that I am more creative. My natural abilities are starting to blossom because I have time to nurture them. I am finding that I have support from my family and friends because I'm not trying to do everything by myself. I am learning to enjoy the process of living instead of constantly pursuing some new accomplishment.

How different today is from the day in front of the mirror. I'm learning to live a life that is rewarding and fulfilling. I know that my family is committed to me, for they have proved it over and over during this time of healing. My natural abilities and expertise are being woven together to help others become healthier.

Have I arrived? No. Do I have down days? Yes. Am I a failure because of that? NO! I have the opportunity to get up, refocus, and keep moving. Progressing through the process of getting healthier means fewer downtimes. The time between down days is longer. The severity of downtimes is less. That is progress and that is good. I've not arrived, but I'm sure improving.

I know that I am blessed and healthy. But I do not hold a private lease on this blessing of health. It is available to everyone. It is possible to succeed where failure has always prevailed. Health is not a mysterious prize that only a few can obtain. *Health is a lifestyle available to anyone—including* YOU.

Are you ready? Let's take the next step.

CHAPTER TWO

What Is Wellness?

As I got up today, I pushed the button to turn off the alarm clock. I pushed a button to turn on the lights as I got out of bed. I juiced my oranges in my electric juicer while my whole-wheat bread browned in the electric toaster. Forest headed off in our car, which will quickly transport him to his high-tech office. I sat at my computer and pushed buttons on the keyboard to write a book. I pushed a button to start my little space heater. When the phone rang, I let the answering machine get it. Then I pushed another button to retrieve the message. What an example of our modern society—*instant* anything and everything!

As a society we have become accustomed to pushing buttons in order to have our needs met—*now*. We don't like to wait. In fact, most of us refuse to wait. Fast food is picked up in the "fast" lane. We deposit our checks in the "express" lane. We order the "daily special" at lunch to minimize our wait. America's refusal to wait has spawned entire industries. From fast food to microwaves to express check-ins to mail-order catalogs to home deliveries, we are a society that wants our needs met instantly.

INSTANT HEALTH

We have transferred that demand to health as well. When we have a temperature and don't feel well, we expect the doctor to give us a pill or prescription (our health button) that will instantly remove the problem and give us back our health. If that doctor won't cooperate, we simply find another, more understanding professional.

What do we do when we find we have a weight problem? We search for a pill, drink, or formula that, when taken, will provide instant weight loss. I recently read that Americans spend more in a year on weight-loss programs than it would cost to feed all of Somalia for a decade.

If our health buttons are truly producing "instant health," why do we have the most significant health-care crisis in this country's history? Is it possible that instant buttons don't work in the area of health? Why, that could never be . . . could it?

One thing I had to learn during my time of healing, which is still continuing, is that health is a process. It's not instant. A process has steps, and each step must be taken in order for the process to be performed. In our culture we have become accustomed to collapsing time frames that make a process seem instant. Our modern washing machines are a far cry from a woman pounding clothes against a rock along a river. Although we can collapse some time frames in the healing process, we still need to take each step, one at a time, in order for health to occur.

The United States has become preoccupied with being sick and overweight. We are continually looking for the proverbial "Fountain of Health and Skinniness." Each person who claims to have found the "magical cure" for these problems is quickly spotlighted, until the next hero emerges. We keep hoping that someone will find that magical pill, cream, or drink that will heal our sickness and eliminate our excess weight.

Time after time, the promised magical cure fails us. After a while we begin to think that we must be the failure and not the magical cure. We begin to perceive that we must be destined to be sick and overweight. Then we begin to believe that our conditions are normal and just the way things are. Isn't everybody we know just like us? Aren't they sick? Aren't they a little overweight? Our problems become normal and acceptable. We begin to accept that normalcy as our new standard of measurement.

SICKNESS VERSUS WELLNESS

If in fact there is an option of health and balanced weight instead of sickness and excess weight, why does that option elude so many Americans? Most of us feel that we already know the difference between sickness and wellness. We are well read on sickness. We talk about it all the time—at home, at work, at the doctor's office. We know what sickness is. Just ask us!

Most of us would say that sickness is not feeling well. Isn't that interesting? That would be like saying that being hot is not being cold. To gain a working knowledge of these two key terms, we must define them more precisely than merely using their opposites.

So, what is sickness? Sickness comes from the root word *sick*, which, according to Webster's unabridged dictionary, means:

a disordered or weakened condition in general, afflicted with disease.

A simple way to remember our focus for disease is to see the word this way: as dis-ease. Dis-ease is when our body is not at ease. When our body is at ease we tend to be healthy. That really is a very simple concept. Two of Webster's definitions for *dis-ease* help us further our understanding. Interestingly, both include the word *health*.

Dis-ease is a condition in which bodily health is seriously attacked, deranged, or impaired. Dis-ease is any departure from the state of health, presenting marked symptoms.

How does the FBI teach their agents to identify counterfeit money? They let the agents handle "real" money. These agents handle the real stuff for so long that they can usually recognize the counterfeit immediately upon contact. Why? *They know the real stuff.*

I believe that part of our problem in attaining health in North America is that we focus on the dis-ease (the counterfeit money) and have failed to understand health (the real stuff). It is time to focus on health and how to obtain health instead of on how to suppress sickness.

NORMAL MAY NOT BE NORMAL

Do you know what it means to be healthy? What is normal, typical, or average for most Americans in the area of health is a far cry from any definition of optimal health. Our nutritionist, Dr. Peter Petropulos, made an interesting comment on this topic. He said,

> "Many patients present themselves to me with what they consider to be 'normal' physical complaints that they do not feel are important (headaches, acid indigestion, menstrual cramping, etc.). *It is of the utmost importance to realize that the body does not produce symptoms of any degree unless it is expending distress of some sort.* The body is not in the business of troubling you for no reason. If you have a symptom, something is wrong and it needs to be addressed. Symptoms are the body's method of drawing attention to its needs."

How many of us perceive symptoms to be an annoying problem that must be quieted, masked, or ignored? How often I had ignored my stress symptoms of tiredness, upset stomach, constipation, and tension headaches! However, unresolved symptoms have an amazing way of "getting even"—they become chronic illnesses, diseases, or other major crises in our lives. Mine nearly killed me. One way or another our body demands to have its symptoms acknowledged. We are the ones who determine when and how we will acknowledge those symptoms.

Being at the brink of death caused me to acknowledge my symptoms and accept the fact that I had a problem. Learning to recognize these symptoms early on as warning signs is key to developing overall health. The alternative is to allow the symptoms to become a crisis or a more severe dis-ease.

Let's take a look at a few of the ailments that so many of us have come to accept as normal. If all we hear from the media is that these ailments are normal, we have no way of knowing that we have options. Through experience, observation, and reading, our family has found that many commonly accepted health problems have their roots in diet, lifestyle, and lack of exercise. We no longer accept "normal" ailments as normal.

Contrary to popular belief, a headache is not caused by a deficiency in aspirin. Neither is acid indigestion a symptom of an antacid shortage. Taking aspirin or antacids is similar to placing a cork in a crying baby's mouth. The noises may go away, but in time the cork will pop.

Have you ever thought you had a "normal" headache? There is no such thing as a "normal" headache. My "normal" afternoon tension headache left for good after I learned how to cleanse and rebuild my body.

What about depression, mood swings, memory loss, inability to concentrate or focus? Does that sound like the old me (and maybe the current you)? Chuck Bates, in his book *Immunity, Mental Health and Essential Fatty Acids*, addresses the link between food allergies and various emotional disorders. What many people consider to be abnormal mental health may be a sign of neurologic stress from food allergies. As I addressed my food allergies, one of the most significant changes I noticed was my loss of anger. All of a sudden my husband and daughter were less irritating. I found myself less angry and less depressed. Our circumstances seemed to become more manageable. I learned that certain foods would trigger anger and depression. That knowledge helped me free myself from what seemed to be an ironclad bondage to uncontrollable emotions.

Did you know that halitosis (more commonly known as bad breath) can be a classic symptom of intestinal congestion and toxicity? Did you know that bad body odor has more to do with your overall health than with which deodorant soap you use? We have found that our bodies now have a sweet smell without the use of perfumes or deodorant soaps. Society's odor problems have created huge industries that are in business to mask our state of deterioration.

Did you know that sinus and ear infections, chronic postnasal drip, and recurring oral lesions (canker sores, fever blisters, etc.) can be classic signs of poor nutrition and toxicity (internal poisons in the body)? Infections are the body's way of saying it has a dis-ease from the presence of microorganisms. We can't see microorganisms. We *can* see or experience the infection. The infection is another of those warning signs we try to suppress instead of determining its source.

Some nutritionists have noted that acne is a skin infection that indicates poor immunity, liver congestion, and malnutrition. Psoriasis and eczema are also symptoms of metabolic imbalances in the body. My skin was one of the first areas of my body to reflect change. As my diet improved and my health improved, my skin began to glow.

Many people have commented that their sore throats, headaches, and skin problems are due to environmental factors. Environmental allergies can be greatly decreased, if not eliminated, by proper diet and supplementation. We can work on eliminating environmental toxins, and we must. We can also develop our body's defense system to deal with, and fight off, those toxins.

Many muscle pains and arthritic conditions can be reduced or eliminated with dietary changes. Toxic build-up of waste products in the muscles greatly inhibits the proper function of the muscular system and leads to inflammation and pain. Helping the body clear its natural detoxification pathways can lead to improved muscular functioning in the body.

Cold hands and feet due to poor circulation can be very responsive to nutritional work. Fingernails that crack, peel, or split can often benefit from good nutrition. Our culture, instead, develops an industry of artificial nails to replace our cracked, split nails. We turn up the heat to warm our cold bodies. It is exciting to have natural, warm hands with natural, nice nails.

The lungs are a source of numerous complaints ranging from asthma to chronic bronchitis to pneumonia. These symptoms result from an inherent weakness of the lungs in the face of stress. Often, food allergies are the direct cause of the weakened lungs. Lung ailments may also be due to poor immune system functioning. As a result of poor diet, the immune system is depleted of necessary nutrients and therefore unable to combat daily intrusions. The lungs are also a primary target of inhaled toxins from the environment.

The heart beats about seventy-two times per minute, or thirty-six million times per year, without rest or sleep. The work it performs in one day is equivalent to lifting about one ton to a height of seventy-five feet. Obviously, the heart needs good nutrition, or fuel, to do its work! Poor nutrition could be a major source of the overwhelming increase in heart surgery and heart malfunction. It is interesting to note that, in spite of our advanced medical techniques and "improved diets," heart disease is still on the rise.

Ulcers, gastritis, acid indigestion, and other digestive symptoms can be the body's way of noting its need for additional nutrients. The liver and gallbladder are sources of many complaints. The liver is the primary detoxifying organ in the body and the main organ of defense, after the intestinal tract. When our trash cans are full in our home, we empty the trash. We don't keep adding trash and then get upset when it overflows. However, when our body is overflowing with trash we get upset and pop an antacid to calm it down.

Colitis, constipation, irritable bowel syndrome, diverticulitis, and hemorrhoids are extremely common in our day. Many of these symptoms are improved by good nutrition. One lady told me she had regular bowels—once a week. Did you know that regular bowels means a bowel movement after every major meal? Did you know that regularity can be achieved without the regular use of laxatives?

PMS (premenstrual syndrome), menopausal symptoms, and infertility are common problems. They are often triggered by malnutrition and constant allergy exposure. How many family fights and professional conflicts are triggered by women with these problems? Chemicals can camouflage the symptoms, but something causes these eruptions. PMS is a thing of the past for me.

A wonderful example of treating cancer with nutrition is presented in Anne Frähm's book, *A Cancer Battle Plan*. After exhausting every traditional medical approach to cancer, Anne found herself dying. In a last-ditch effort to heal herself of cancer she tried a nutritional route. Today, she is alive and healthy.

Many other diseases have been positively affected by nutrition. In my discussions with nutritionists and holistic health practitioners, I am continually amazed at the variety of dis-eases and health problems that are affected. For example, arthritic conditions have been known to improve by eliminating nightshade foods: peppers, tomatoes, and eggplant, among others. Respiratory conditions have been know to improve by eliminating wheat and dairy products. Anemia often responds to the correct supplementation and a diet rich in dark leafy green vegetables and sea vegetables.

Autoimmune diseases, such as lupus, multiple sclerosis, Raynaud's syndrome, scleroderma, and vasculitis, are often helped by eliminating toxic cleaning, laundry, and skin products, while increasing dosages of supplements and foods containing vitamins E and C. Omega-3 and other fatty acids (primrose oil, fish oil, flaxseed oil, etc.) can also be helpful.

One known key to addressing candidiasis is a diet free of sugar, yeast, and mold. Supplementing with vitamins A, B_6, C, copper, iron, magnesium, selenium, and zinc can also be helpful. Bowel irregularities, such as constipation and colitis, can definitely be helped by consuming fewer processed foods and more fruits, vegetables, whole grains, and beans. Increasing the consumption of water is also critical. PMS can often be minimized by reducing the consumption of dairy products, caffeine-containing foods, and refined sugars. Twice as much vegetable protein should be consumed than animal protein.

Many other common ailments can be positively affected by

diet and supplementation. Working with a quality health-care provider can help you understand these options. Melvyn R. Werbach, M.D., in *Nutrition Influences of Illness*, discusses one hundred common ailments and how nutrition can affect them.[1]

I, and many others, am alive and well today because I learned about wellness and how to bring it about naturally through nutrition, lifestyle, and exercise. Traditional medicine had not been able to offer any workable solutions to my health problems. It became apparent that I had to take responsibility for my own health. Doctors and other health-care providers that I selected became a resource in my overall health plan.

So, if all of these common ailments are not indications of wellness, they must be symptoms of sickness. As we pursue wellness, we begin to consider these symptoms as warning signs instead of annoyances to suppress.

TAKING RESPONSIBILITY

One key difference I see, on a regular basis, between sick people and well people is in the area of responsibility. Well people take the responsibility for their health instead of being the victim of their dis-ease. When I accepted that I had a problem with my health and decided to correct it, I took my first step toward becoming healthy.

We accept this philosophy in the area of alcohol and sobriety. When people admit they have a drinking problem and decide to live each day being sober, we applaud them. However, in the area of sickness, when we are in a crisis, we decide that someone else must heal us. We embrace the belief that we are the victim of dis-ease. Being a victim removes the responsibility of a solution from our shoulders and places it on someone else. We seek out

> *A key attribute of a person seeking health is that he or she acknowledges symptoms as warning signs, not as annoyances to suppress.*

that someone to heal us of our problem. We lead the life of a victim.

If we watched an alcoholic behave this way, we would say that he or she was being irresponsible. Are we not, in fact, being irresponsible in the area of our own health? Few people accept that they have a health problem and decide to live each day being healthy. I have personally never met a recovering, dying diseased person who did not take responsibility for his or her own health. There is freedom in acknowledging a problem and deciding to deal with it. That freedom has helped bring me and my family health.

HEALTHY BENEFITS . . . MMMM GOOD!

Having walked the path of illness, high-level stress, suicide attempts, and severe depression, I know what it's like to be healthy. And it's worth every perceived sacrifice that I made. There is no comparison between where I am today and where I was when I was in the pit of sickness. We have developed a lifestyle of health that has given us a much larger return than our investment. That return can be measured in very real benefits.

First, we have more *time*. Being sick takes time. It affects your personal time, your work schedule, your school schedule, and your social time. We have virtually eliminated the downtime caused by the "normal" flu bug, cold, sniffles, etc. We haven't had those ailments in several years. When we get a minor symptom in those areas, we immediately fight it and build up our bodies with good food, regular sleep, and supplements.

We wake up each day feeling rested and ready to go. When we need to work extra hours, we have the energy to do it. However, we make sure the time demand is temporary. When that demand ends, we go back to our normal routine, instead of allowing the increased demand to become our new routine.

Second, becoming healthy emotionally has helped us develop *emotional stability*. Depression and mood swings are like a pair of glasses that distort every thought and feeling. It is virtually impossible to be stable when your "glasses" present a world that is always out of focus and tilted. Being able to clearly distinguish feelings and needs has helped to produce a sense of relaxed peace and well-being. I have become more acutely aware of how unpeaceful and uptight sick people are. The most peaceful and relaxed people I know are those who are pursuing health in a significant manner.

Third, mental health produces *the ability to think clearly and behave consistently*. Confusion, which is a cousin to depression, can easily distort our thinking and behavior. We have noticed a big difference between our daughter and other children her age. Children with poor eating habits, irregular rest, and infrequent exercise tend to have a lack of focus, an inability to concentrate, and erratic behavior.

As a family, we are able to focus and finish a job that we have determined to do. That has significantly affected our daughter's ability to focus, her performance at school, and her overall behavior. Forest has been able to excel in his job due to his increased ability to focus and follow through.

Fourth, our *physical benefits* are almost too numerous to mention. Forest and I both lost weight. This was a secondary benefit for us; the primary issue was for me to live and become functional. However, we both lost over forty pounds. It was interesting to us that we both lost that weight in our "fat" areas. For me, that was my thighs and hips. For Forest, it was his abdomen and rear. What a delight to see that part of us leave and not come back. We have not had to focus on maintaining our weight. It has remained within about five pounds in either direction for over four years, without a fight from us.

We have watched so many friends lose weight and fight to keep it off, only to see it come back again and again. When the body is in balance, with the correct nutrition and exercise, weight control becomes almost automatic. We have learned to understand what our body needs (versus craves) and respond accordingly. The result is a stable weight and overall health.

We now sleep well. I never knew that insomnia could be related to diet. We now know that when we feel tired after our normal amount of sleep, we have a symptom that we need to examine. It is refreshing to know that our sleep time will be spent resting and not tossing and turning.

Our skin and eyes look healthy. One of the first indicators that a person has cleansed his or her body is a bright, clear complexion and bright, clear eyes. This person truly begins to glow. No cosmetic can duplicate that look. That glow is inner beauty shining out through healthy skin and eyes. We have experienced that. When we notice our skin or eyes looking dull, we know we have another symptom to examine. When we see morning bags under our eyes, we know that our body is carrying baggage it should not be carrying. We have learned how to unpack that baggage and clean our body. Yes, this is an ongoing process; it is a *lifestyle* of health.

We have also learned how to create a physically clean home that is a haven. I'm talking about more than dust and dirt. We have learned how to remove many of the chemicals from the air, carpet, and our household cleaners. The result is a home that does not aggravate environmental allergies or sensitivities.

Last but not least, we have realized significant *financial returns*. Anne Frähm, author of *A Cancer Battle Plan*, says it best: "I spent more than 250,000 dollars dying with cancer and I spent less than two thousand dollars getting well."

We are more productive in our jobs, and our finances reflect that increased productivity. We are not stuck in a job in order to keep our health insurance. We have freedom and mobility both professionally and financially. Yes, it costs money to eat healthfully and to pursue health. But the costs pale in the light of current health-care costs for degenerative dis-eases or death. In addition, every dollar our family spends on our health has been an investment that has brought us a return.

Does this mean you should stop any physical or psychological treatments you are currently taking? Does being healthier mean the total absence of all problems? No, to both questions. Getting healthier means starting right where you are. It means finding qualified health-care providers to help you learn about your options. Once you are aware of your options and have a quality team of professionals, you can begin to develop a game plan. One step at a time, you can begin to move. Each step of improvement will affect your whole person.

Becoming healthier mentally impacts a person's emotional responses. Physical healing affects a person's energy level. Each area impacts the others. We are a whole, integrated package. The process of becoming healthy must address the whole package of a person in order to be effective in the long term.

Wellness or sickness? Each of us chooses our preoccupation. Each preoccupation produces a return. The good news is that you can choose. Want to make a change? I heartily recommend seeking wellness and all of its many benefits!

Part Two
Food for Thought

CHAPTER THREE

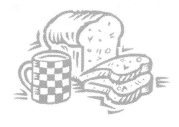

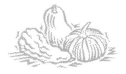

Prepare for Change

Many people know they need to change their diets and improve their health. Many of these people even want to change. So, they follow this diet and that diet. They work at controlling their food cravings. Yet, repeatedly, they fail. They get only so far in their change, and then they fail. The roller coaster ride of starting and failing, starting and failing, causes them to see themselves as failures destined for sickness and excess weight.

My heart goes out to those people. It is devastating to try to do something, only to see our efforts end in failure. The old tapes pop into our mind. "What did I do wrong this time?" "What is wrong with me?" Failure turns into discouragement and a sense of hopelessness. Each new attempt toward health is exciting. Yet, so often we revert to our old behavior, dis-eases, and weight. How do we sabotage ourselves in this area of our lives?

Most people have talked to health-care practitioners, gone to seminars, and read books on the subject of health. Most of those resources tell us what to eat and what not to eat, what to do and what not to do. So why does America continue to face an escalating health-care crisis? Why aren't we getting any healthier?

PREGNANT WITH HEALTH

Let's look at the analogy of giving birth to a child. When Forest and I thought about having a child, we didn't automatically become pregnant. Our thinking about a child didn't cause me to become pregnant.

When I did become pregnant, I didn't have our baby the next day. It took time for our baby to grow, develop, and be born. During that time I went to classes, saw my doctor, and read books on childbirth and parenting. I learned everything I could. All of that information didn't make me pregnant, but it did help me prepare for the different phases of pregnancy, birth, and parenting.

Health and wellness operate in much the same manner. All

> *Become pregnant with health.*

of the doctors, books, and classes in the world won't make you healthy. Health is born when you get a revelation in your heart that *you* want to be healthy. When that revelation gets embedded in your heart and mind, it sprouts a life of its own, and you become pregnant with health.

Being pregnant with health doesn't mean that you have the physical manifestation of health. Did I have a physical baby the day I got pregnant? No. Although the full manifestation took time, the process had begun and was alive. A strong, burning desire for health will produce health.

Doctors will tell you that the desire to live is a critical component for a terminally ill patient. If the person does not have a desire to live, the person will die. Being healthy requires a strong desire to be healthy. Without that desire, all of the information on health will never be enough to make you healthy.

Pregnancy is designed to be a time of preparation. Learning to change what we eat is part of the preparation for getting healthy, but it isn't where health begins. Health takes on life with the desire to be healthy and the revelation about what health really is. As that desire burns inside you, you will naturally begin to prepare yourself for the necessary changes in your life. Something is different inside you: You want to be healthy, not sickly.

WHY PREPARE FOR HEALTH?

Why is preparation so important to the process of getting healthy? Can't we just skip it and move right to the job of eating right and exercising? We want our health right now. We don't want to wait. Why do we have to nickel-and-dime our way through all of this preparation stuff?

We would never hire a builder to build us a house without a blueprint. Why? He might build a house we didn't like. The house might be too expensive. We would think a builder was ridiculous to even suggest building without any plans. Those plans represent our house. They are our imagined house until we have the real thing.

Preparing for health is a critical part of the process of our becoming healthy. That preparation is the picture of our desired health that we don't yet have.

To prepare for health, we must first become aware of our mind-sets regarding food. Food is a very basic part of our life. We celebrate with food. Food is withheld to punish us. We share food with friends, family, and even enemies. We eat when we are sad, glad, and mad. Day or night, we eat for all kinds of reasons. Since food is part of every area of our life, changing what we eat is a very major alteration for all of us.

Most health-care providers offer patients information on the necessary food choices. People know they need to make these changes. Yet, so often no one helps them mentally and emotionally prepare to live with those food choices. It is crucial that people take the time to understand why they eat the way they do. This is a crucial step to produce long-lasting food changes.

Our mind-sets represent our habits. Our food beliefs and thoughts become our daily, automatic habits. Many of us are not even aware of those thoughts or beliefs. Eating is a habit. Little do we think about what we eat. We just eat.

My computer is preprogrammed with certain automatic

options. Whenever I choose, I can override those automatic options. However, they will instantly apply the next time I use that program. A temporary override never replaces the automatic programming. To replace the defaults, I have to reprogram the default part of the software.

Our habits are similar to computer defaults. They automatically operate until we reprogram them. We can override old habits anytime we want, but if we don't reprogram them we will, without thinking, revert to our old, automatic habits.

We have automatic habits in every area of our lives. This is especially true for food. We can override these habits with regulated food choices for a time. However, when the diet is over or we encounter extra stress or various temptations, etc., without thinking, we revert right back to our automatic habits. Why? Our automatic habits, or mental mind-sets, regarding food have never been reprogrammed.

> *Our mind has an automatic pilot regarding food.*

Most people never take the time to look at their habits, or mind-sets, regarding food. They simply try to carry out new rules, formulas, or diets. They think that maybe this formula or that diet will be just the right one for them. Their automatic habits stand by ready to sabotage their efforts. Their mind-sets don't change and, consequently, that diet also fails.

Mental, emotional, and physical breakdowns teach a person many things. Mine taught me that my mind was as sick as my body. Books and resources told me how to make my body healthy. Few told me how to make my mind healthy. Even fewer helped me understand the connection between mind and body. How could I make my mind healthy? My mind needed to be as healthy as my body.

Could I ever find the kind of "food" that would make my mind functional? My mind didn't need to get smarter or to gather more information on health. Wisdom was my goal. I wanted to customize this health information for me. I wanted this "health stuff" to work for me. I wanted to get my act together. I wanted my mind and body to function together instead of fighting each other. I wanted to be a functional person and live with a sense of purpose.

Several times Forest has jokingly said I should be a brain in a jar without a body. Although at times that would be convenient, I have yet to see anyone successfully live that way. Our mind resides inside our body and directs it. Our body transports our mind to where it needs to go. They are highly dependent on each other. Mental health cannot be overlooked in the process of getting healthy.

Our mind and body work together.

OUR MIND: THE HEART OF WHO WE ARE

Our mind reflects how we think and directs our actions. We can do whatever we make up our mind to do. We use our mind to remember. Life's experiences are contained in our memory. With our mind we think and form our opinions. Our thoughts give expression to our desires and fears. With our mind we store information and develop skills and abilities.

This quick look at the mind's role shows us that our mind-sets affect our food intake. Our mind tells us what we think about food and what to eat. When we decide to eat some particular food, that is exactly what we do.

We remember eating candy at Christmas and cake on our birthday. Our mind reminds us that we feel better when we eat after someone yells at us. We select restaurants based on our memories and opinions. We shop for food based on how we were taught to shop. Our mind plays a vital role in our selection of food.

With our memories, thoughts, and knowledge, we form mind-sets, which form our habits. These habits are like mental highways. Habits are how we mentally go about doing what we do. Knowingly or unknowingly, our automatic habits affect

Our mind makes our food choices.

every area of our life.

My own breakdown was like having a mental earthquake. Remember the media coverage of the 1994 Los Angeles earthquake? We saw pictures of highways and roads ripped and torn apart. The vehicles on the highways were left hanging or destroyed. That is a vivid picture of how my mind felt after my breakdown. I couldn't clearly go from one thought to another. Without coherent thoughts I couldn't figure out how I felt. I was as shocked as any earthquake victim.

You may not experience a mental and emotional breakdown, but you probably have some shaky ground in your mind. For example, do you think you must be healthy because you don't look sick? Does everybody get healthy the same way? Is healthy eating complicated and expensive? Should food choices always feel comfortable? Can you get healthy all by yourself? Is it okay to eat whatever you want as long as you exercise enough? Are you so healthy it doesn't really matter what you eat? A yes to any of those questions reflects shaky ground that could give way to disaster.

How can such a disaster be prevented? Or if the disaster has already happened, how can we recover from it? In either case, a person needs to clean house. We need to clean up our false mind-sets and poor habits. A healthy mind builds a healthy body.

CLEANING HOUSE

The first step my nutritionist took me through was a cleanse. During a cleanse, a person eats very simple food or drinks fresh juices, or a combination of the two. The purpose is to help the body eliminate toxins—poisons stored throughout the body that cause dis-ease.

A healthy body assimilates food. I had to clean my body of years of accumulated garbage before it could begin assimilating healthy food.

An old house (versus a new house that has never been occupied) usually needs some work. You would not move your good furniture into a dirty, broken house without doing some cleaning.

You might even hire professionals to help clean the carpets or refinish the hardwood floors. You might repaint or add fixtures. You might redo the plumbing and electrical systems or add extra lighting. If you needed more functional space, you would hire a contractor to help you remodel.

Cleanses eliminate garbage.

After all of those activities, and probably others, you would be ready to live in your wonderfully clean and remodeled house. You never planned to spend your entire life cleaning and remodeling your house or wallowing in the mess. Your goal was to make your house livable. You wanted to move in and use the house for all of its many purposes: protection, storage, hospitality, sleeping, etc.

That is just what a cleanse is like. My nutritionist represented my contractor. I brought in other system specialists as we reached that part of my house or my body. My electrical system, or the energy system of my body, was reworked. The immune, adrenal, digestive, and eliminatory systems were cleansed. We cleaned out the liver and gallbladder, which hold the body's trash. The goal of my physical cleanse was to build a healthy body.

A mental cleanse is just as critical as a physical one. Your beliefs are examined during a mental cleanse. The next four chapters will walk you through a mental cleanse on food and health. As you identify your not-so-healthy mind-sets, you will have the opportunity to replace them with new, healthy mind-sets.

As you finish your mental cleanse, you will become better equipped to make healthier food choices. Just as with your own house, you don't "deep-clean" every day or even every month. Most of us regularly clean our house. Keeping our mind and body clean is an ongoing process, not a one-time event. Each time we clean, we get better and better at it.

Denial is an unhealthy mind-set. Many people operate in the realm of denial when it comes to food. They deny that food affects them. They want to eat whatever they feel like eating whenever they feel like eating it. Food choices have nothing to

51

do with their health problem. The relationship between food and health is denied.

When a health problem occurs, they want to pop a pill and have the problem disappear. Someone else should fix their problem. It's not their fault that they are sick. Why can't the doctors give them the right medicine? People in denial expect somebody else to do something to take care of them.

I operated in denial just like everybody else. It seemed impossible that my stressful lifestyle and diet had affected my health. My denials were as strong as any cancer tumor. Besides, I ate "better" than most of my friends, didn't I? It was difficult to admit that my lifestyle and food choices had contributed to my sickness. Admitting that meant I had to change my lifestyle and food choices. That made me, not someone else, responsible for my sickness and my health. I had to face some heavy doses of truth.

> *Denial is an unhealthy mind-set.*

Another unhealthy mind-set is our unwillingness to admit that health has a cost. We want to be healthy and yet do whatever we want to do, however we want to do it. Discipline seems too high a price for health. Let's eat what we want today and pay the health cost later.

Our world is based on credit. Tomorrow's money pays for today's wants. We have learned how to borrow whatever we need so that we can immediately satisfy our desires. Credit is so easy. It is so much simpler to pay $200 a month for a car than $15,000 up front.

Eventually the bills come due. Bill paying is never as much fun as spending. Too much borrowing produces a problem. We soon learn that we are in debt and a poor credit risk. Our financial problems build. The debt becomes too massive and bankruptcy bails us out. Our financial problems have grown into a crisis.

We use the same philosophy with our health. Today we eat whatever we want; tomorrow we promise to eat better. No thought is given to the cost of our choices. We borrow our way through life. The bill comes due as dis-ease and sickness: cancer, heart dis-ease, and many other illnesses. The cost of our health problems are mounting into a national crisis of health (make that dis-ease) care.

Poor food choices produce poor health.

Breaking out of debt requires us to take responsibility for our choices and purchases. Impulses must be considered instead of automatically obeyed. We must acknowledge the cost of each choice.

How then do we go about getting cleaned up? Cleaning up my act, so to speak, made the whole issue of health personal. That process was critical to my total health, and I have watched many individuals and families benefit from it. Part 2 of this book, "Food for Thought," will help you clean up your mind. Part 3, "Food for the Body," will help you build a stronger body.

Here are a few of the steps I took during the preparation phase. First, I had to step out of my role of victim and become responsible for my own health. I had to learn that becoming responsible is a process. That meant I had to give myself time to become healthy. It had taken me years to get sick. It would take more than a day or two to get healthy.

Second, I had to decide *why* I wanted to get healthy. The why process makes health information personal and meaningful. No longer could I expect someone else to do what I needed to do. Health professionals could share their expertise with me, but I was the one who had to make the changes.

Third, I had to learn to keep everything simple. Simple steps, one at a time, had to be taken. This process had to work for me and my family, not someone else. I couldn't do something just because it worked for someone else. It had to work for me. My process had to be simple enough to work for me right where I was.

Fourth, I had to find ways to encourage myself. I surrounded myself with friends and family who wanted to see me healthy. I thank God that I had a husband who was supportive of me during my healing process. He was my best friend, biggest defender, and strongest ally. You need that kind of physical and emotional support as you mentally and physically cleanse and rebuild your health.

Fifth, I had to learn to acknowledge my progress. Some sick people are negative and critical, especially of themselves. I had to learn to see my progress instead of just my mistakes and failures. Learn to focus on your progress. Let unimportant things go by the wayside so that you can do what is really important.

LIVING HEALTHY!

The best part of getting healing for me is where I am today. I have rebuilt my life out of near death. My body is healthier than ever before. Creativity is helping me develop recipes for wonderfully healthy, tasty food. My computer and business skills are helping me develop a business that moves other people toward health. Most important, I am enjoying my life as never before.

A short time ago it occurred to me that I had entered a new season. No longer was I just cleansing and rebuilding my body. I had moved into the phase of healthy living! Living in my clean house—my body and mind—is exciting! My body and mind are working together. I have laid the foundation and paid the price, and now I am experiencing the rewards.

As you read the chapters on "Food for Thought," please don't belittle their significance. This is the foundation that will help you successfully implement the "Food for the Body" chapters. Cleaning your mind will lay the groundwork for your overall health. Practice healthy food choices. Continue to live each day as best as you can. One day, you too will notice that you are living as a whole, healthy person.

Your preparation for change along with your actual changes will help you become *food smart* in every sense of the term.

CHAPTER
FOUR

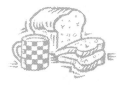

Change Is a Process

You might be saying, "I've been here before. Every time I try something new I end up failing. What's wrong with me? Why doesn't it work for me?" You have raised a key issue.

Change, by its very definition, means to grow, move, or transfer from one place to another. Change requires movement or action. That movement is a process. Many people see health as an event and they miss the process.

"It has taken time for you to get to where you are, and it will take time to get to a different place." Being a driver, first child, German, type-A person, I hate statements like that. I want to see a change occur instantly, if not sooner. It has taken me years to appreciate the fact that permanent, healthy changes take time.

Time and habits are the tools we use to build or destroy our lives. Changing habits takes time—approximately twenty-one days. A desired habit takes less time to maintain than to build. The initial time is an investment.

If you want to become healthier, it becomes important to realize that you need to change some habits. Guess what? *You* get to decide how quickly you make those changes. You can move quickly, or you can take your time. An intense program is usually necessary when you are on the brink of dying. More time can be taken when your condition is less critical. That is okay. You decide how quickly you want to reach your goal.

> *One reason people fail to get healthy is that they don't prepare to change.*

This chapter looks at steps contained in the process of getting healthy. The number-one reason for failure is not preparing to change. Our lifestyle is who we are. Changing basic components of our lifestyle changes part of who we are. That kind of change is not one to shrug off lightly.

Look at food. Changing what we eat affects a very large part of our lifestyle. It affects how we shop, how we cook, where we eat, and many other aspects of our life.

My goal is for you to succeed in your health changes. I want to share with you what causes people to repeatedly fail. Break the failure barrier. Begin to experience real health and weight control, perhaps for the first time in your life.

TAKING OWNERSHIP

When we went to our nutritionist, he offered us something no other traditional health-care practitioner had offered us. Rather than offer me a pill or an instant remedy, he explained *why* I had the problems I had and where the probable root was for each of my major symptoms. He offered me an alternative that would take time but would bring results. It all depended on my willingness to learn a new way of caring for my body. My wellness became dependent upon my willingness to be responsible for my own health.

I could no longer blame the doctor, my parents, some undefined stress, my job, my boss, my finances, my husband, my child, or anyone or anything else. I was sick and I was the one who had to get well. That goal was now my responsibility. I had to take a long, hard look at what had brought me to the brink of death. My nutritionist helped me place the proverbial mirror in front of myself.

My sickness had not happened by accident. Years of patterns, habits, and beliefs—eating, thinking, and emotional in nature—had shaped my current state of sickness. By the time we finished our first interview with our nutritionist, I had become aware of these facts. No longer could I remain blind to my involvement in creating my problem. I finally accepted ownership of it.

Healthy people accept responsibility for their own health.

As I listen to people talk about getting healthy, I hear many responses. Some people say, "We really eat healthily" or "We are healthy." A few minutes later they might mention taking their children to the doctor or guiltily talk about what they ate for lunch. I find these people have no clear definition of health. Their definition of "health food" is any packaged food with the word *natural* somewhere on the label. Do they really understand health? How can they know if they are healthy if they don't know what health is?

Some people say, "I could never eat like you do. I have to work, and I just don't have time." Later those people talk about being home for days, if not weeks, with the common flu. Where did their time go?

Some people say, "I can't afford to eat health food. It costs too much." Those same people talk about their doctor bills and the high cost of medical insurance and prescription drugs. They also bring home bags of groceries of expensive "snack" items. Where did their money go?

Other people say, "I don't know how to cook. If it's not in a box or a freezer bag, I can't cook it." These same people are often highly trained professionals with advanced training and education in their chosen professions. Is the issue that they can't cook or that they don't want to cook?

Other people comment, "You are really radical in your approach to eating. I would never want to do what you do." These people are often the chronic complainers. They complain about their sickness, their doctor, the price of medicine, and almost everything else. Do they prefer complaining to being healthy?

WHICH ONE ARE YOU?

I have observed that most people fall into one of the following categories.

1. They are a victim of their circumstances and feel powerless to change anything. *These are victims.*
2. They acknowledge they have a problem, but they don't want to exert any effort to change. *These are the "yes-but" people.*
3. They accept that they have a problem and they choose to address it. *These are the winners!*

The first category describes people who are victims to their circumstances or to other people. Victims blame everybody else for their problems. They change doctors at the drop of a hat while trying every new fad and every new "miracle" diet. Diets are ineffective for them. They complain about their medical costs. Hopelessness runs their life. Victims are defensive, hopeless, and negative.

These people do not believe there is any hope. Trapped in their pit of sickness and hopelessness, they barely exist.

At a recent seminar, a young person came to me regarding her mother. Her mother, a highly depressed person, had not wanted to come to my presentation. She had just been released from a mental hospital. Many of her symptoms seemed to be getting worse. She blamed everyone else for her problems and refused to seek help. Beside herself, the young woman cried, "What can I do?"

I have found a few techniques that might help both of those people. As I look back at myself when I was the most depressed, I notice several similar patterns to the above situation. I didn't want to be around people. People always asked me, "How are you doing?" That question really annoyed me. Knowing the answer to that question would mean that I had already helped myself. I would have told them if it was any different from the last time they saw me. Besides, I thought, *It's none of your business!* I came to hate and resent the question "How are you doing?" That question is not effective. I no longer ask sick people how they are doing.

So, what can be said? Often, I say nothing. Let the person know that you love him or her. Help the person in any way possible. Take healthy, tasty meals to the person. Send notes of encouragement. Live your life as an example that it is possible to overcome great obstacles with faith and effort.

I also suggested to this young person that she not try to change her mom. Until the mom wants to change, there is not a lot the daughter can do. Changing someone is the definition of a manipulator or controller. Control and manipulation bring their own set of problems.

I encouraged this young woman to show love and support to her mother. She could take her mother to helpful activities, if her mother wanted to go. Accept Mom the way she is. That does not mean that we accept the sickness. We accept the person, not the sickness.

The last suggestion I gave the young person was to work at getting healthy herself. She admitted having many of her mother's symptoms. So often we see how much someone else needs help and we miss how much we need it ourselves. Take your eyes off others long enough to look in the mirror. Are you maybe ignoring your own problems and using others as your excuse to stay sick? You can support and help other people, but the only person you can truly change is *you*.

> *A healthy person changes only himself or herself.*

The second category describes yes-but people. These people agree with all of your suggestions. They attend seminars and agree with everything said. However, when it comes to personal application, they always have a *but*.

My "yes-but" cancels everything I say before the but. For

example, Forest asks me how he looks. I might say, "You look great, but why are you wearing those socks with those pants?" What am I really saying? I am really saying that he doesn't look very good at all. Yes-but people say they want to get healthy. They follow that statement with all of the reasons they can't get healthy. Actually, they don't want to pay the price to be healthy at all.

These yes-but people remind me of a great definition of insanity: Doing the same thing and expecting a new result.

Yes-but people think that, somehow, doing more of their current activity will cause them to get healthier. Their dis-ease will just go away by itself. Isn't that an amazing idea?

The third category describes people who are winners. Rewarding and inspirational people are like sponges. They soak up information. Winners work at understanding their problems. The best they could do has gotten them where they are. They don't like where they are, so they choose to do something about it. These people are winners in every sense of the word.

The fact that you are reading this book says that you are, or can be, a winner. You know that you have a problem. You want to deal with your problem. You are acknowledging that *you* have a problem. That is good. I applaud you! You have taken a giant step toward getting healthy.

Admitting you have a problem is an important step. You have laid the foundation that only you can lay, and you have laid it on rock instead of on sand. Now your efforts will produce results that will stand and not blow over in the face of a storm. So what is your next step?

DON'T PANIC: TAKE TIME

How often I watch people attend a seminar, hear a dynamic speaker, and leave with every book, tape, and piece of information available. They plan to do every step, buy every recommended product, and be totally new by . . . tomorrow. As we read this we think how ridiculous these folks are. Of course, *we* would never do that. Yet how often do we do just that?!

It's your time and your life. You may spend it as you choose.

I was on the brink of death, so I no longer had much time to spend getting well. You have more time when you aren't dying. Close to death or not, don't panic. Panic swallows time in large gulps and leaves nothing to show for it. Panic will not help you better use whatever time you do have.

You can only do what you can do. It is okay to take time and do the best you can.

Take your time and pick your timing. I had a friend come over to me a year ago, during November. In her midthirties, she was on the highest level possible of heart medication, antidepressants, and many other types of medications. She was overweight and suffered from anxiety attacks. After hearing my story she had some questions. She needed to go through a similar cleanse, but didn't know where to start. As we talked, several things became obvious.

"How quickly do I start?" she asked. My first suggestion was that she wait until after the holidays. Her personality type indicated impulsive tendencies. I was convinced, as she is now, that a preholiday start would have caused her to fail. Instead, she took about three months to plan her change. She started that February. Eleven months later, she had lost over thirty pounds. Her medication is history, and she looks great. Did her timing make a difference? It made all the difference between success and failure for her!

Pick your timing and take your time.

A family we know well looked at the results of our health changes and asked how we had achieved them. We shared the process. After weighing the cost of constant family sickness, weight problems, and crying kids, they decided to try something. Getting started is critical. This family spent the next twelve months eliminating sugar from their diet. That was a major step for them. Then, they worked at getting white flour out of their diet.

Soon, the ball began to roll more quickly. Now they have moved much farther along the health process. As a family, they are healthy. They rarely deal with ear infections, chronic respiratory problems, and runny noses. They started slowly, stayed with it, and today they are reaping the harvest of improved health.

You are dealing with your health and your life. Take the time to do what you need to do. Do it right. Take one step at a time. Getting started may seem hard, but that is the first step. Start where you are with one small step. Each step leads to the next. Soon, you will have gone farther than you ever thought possible.

DEFINE YOUR PROBLEM

In the second chapter we talked about symptoms. So often people think that if they just eliminate their symptoms, they will auto-matically be well. I personally have never seen health work that way. This is especially true in the area of weight control. Our family has learned that as we eat the right food our weights stay level, within about five pounds in either direction. This has been true for us for years.

> *Take the time to get started.*

Have you ever known people who picked the dandelion blooms in their lawn and expected that to eliminate the dande-lion problem? Does that sound silly? Everybody knows that dan-delions have deep roots; to eliminate them we have to kill the root. This is just like our health issues. To eliminate dis-ease, we must do more than pick the blooms of symptoms. We must identify and eliminate the dis-ease roots.

During the problem-definition period, I highly recommend that you find a good health-care team to help you zero in on your roots. I probably would not be here today if I had not found the health-care practitioners that I found. If you have no idea where to begin to look, I recommend that you contact HealthQuarters at (719)593-8694. They have produced a booklet of health-care people from throughout the United States. HealthQuarters is a nonprofit organization, dedicated to providing national education and health resources (see appendix F, page 224).

Look at the health of the health-care practitioner. Does he or she seem healthy? So often we forget to observe whether the person giving advice is healthy. If these professionals can't bring health into their own life, how can they help you bring health into yours? Qualified resource people who are personally healthy increase your ability to identify the roots of your dis-ease accurately.

Find a qualified health-care practitioner.

Defining a client's problem was directly, and critically, linked to my success as a business consultant. I learned several ways to obtain that problem's definition.

ASK QUESTIONS

Much of my time was spent asking questions. I asked the same questions of many people. I asked different questions of each person. After a while, a pattern would begin to emerge. The more successful a consultant I became, the better my questioning skills became.

Know-it-all people spend more time telling than asking questions. Don't be a know-it-all with your health-care practitioner. Get your money's worth! Ask questions. Take some time before your appointments to write down every question you can think to ask. Often patients will arrive at a practitioner's office and forget their questions. This is a waste of everybody's time and money.

Learn to ask a lot of questions.

Besides your health-care practitioner, seek out people who "have good fruit" in their lives. The fruit says something about the tree from which it came. Good trees do not produce bad fruit. Bad trees do not consistently produce good fruit. That idea applies in nearly every other area of life. We have learned to look at our trees. My sick body (my fruit) told me something about my diet and lifestyle (the tree). Our impoverished finances (the fruit) told us something about our spending and employment (the tree). Our daughter's behavior (fruit) told us something about our parenting (the tree).

When we had our financial disaster, we sought out people we knew who had good financial fruit in their lives. We asked them every question we could. We watched them, learned from them, and were influenced by them. We applied what we learned, and we now have good fruit in that area of our lives.

Find people who are healthy and ask them questions. Find the common patterns among those people. Learn from their mistakes and their successes. Ask and keep asking questions.

Just as it helps to learn from "good fruit," so it is harmful to hang around "spoiled fruit." Remember the old adage "A rotten apple spoils the whole bunch"? When we have a problem with our health, hanging around sick people will only further depress us. Be very selective of the "fruit" with which you surround yourself. Check out your "fruit basket." Is the fruit sweet and healthy? Is the fruit spoiled? That fruit will affect you. It may be time to clean out your fruit basket.

> *Find people with "good fruit" and learn from them.*

A QUICK REVIEW

Let's review the major keys to help ensure that you break through any barriers you might have. First, it is critical that you prepare for your changes. Your preparation is a key to your success. Second, take responsibility for your problems and your solutions. No one else can do this. Without you leading the process, the process will not happen. Third, become a winner, instead of a victim or a yes-but person. Fourth, don't panic. Take your time and pick your timing. It is your time. Fifth, define your problem as accurately as possible. Go beyond the symptoms and get to the root. Sixth, find a qualified health-care practitioner and build a team to help you in your healing process. Those people may take time to find, but it is well worth the time invested. Last, for this chapter, is to check your fruit. Is it healthy or spoiled? Remember, fruit never falls far from the tree.

Yes, change is a process with many steps. Are you feeling

a little overwhelmed? That's normal. Just remember, you have to take only one step at a time.

Now is the time to look at the next question, "Why bother changing?" The answer to this question is the primary motivator for making changes and the glue that will hold you together during your change process.

CHAPTER FIVE

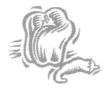

Why Bother?

Have you ever found yourself trying to change, yet somehow ending up right where you started? Does your schedule seem to afford you little, if any, time to even consider changing? Maybe the carrot of health seems dependent on changing too many things all at once. For many of us, the desire to change is there, but the perceived requirements seem to be a little overwhelming. For others, the obsession to do it perfectly keeps us from even trying to do one little part.

Our media-driven society constantly confronts us with images of slender, apparently healthy and successful men and women. Comparing ourselves to those media images, we feel like total failures. Trying to duplicate those images, we buy every trendy fad and product they sell. Time after time this results in failure or, at best, intense stress for us and megasales for the companies.

I decided to break away from the standards of "perfection" provided by the media. My goal was to become the best Cheryl I could be. I can now admire a model, but envy to be like her does not possess me. As I pursue my process of becoming healthy, I am learning that it is okay to be Cheryl. I may never achieve the media's definition of a perfect body. However, I can certainly have a healthy body.

The last several years have seen me speaking to many people through the avenues of books, newsletters, cooking classes, and seminars. As I tell my story, many people begin to hope that just maybe they, too, can become healthy. Often, when they hear the basics of my story, they come to me and say, "Will this really work? Come on, really, really work? Will it work for me?"

Without a doubt it works for me. Will it work for you? Well, that depends on your response to the following statement:

Without a satisfactory answer to the question why? *any price will be too great.*

So many people enter into health changes without adequately answering the question, "Why am I doing this?" As a result, when they find that there is a price to pay to be healthy, they quickly lose interest and quit. The price to change seems too great. You, not someone else, must know why you want to change. Otherwise, any price for health will seem too great.

MAKE YOUR REASONS PERSONAL

In my situation, I knew why I was changing my lifestyle—I was dying. Coming home from the hospital was my change catalyst. I examined my situation. I was overweight. My skin was an itchy, bleeding mess. Meals left me bloated and constipated. Constipation was chronic, as was my overall inability to adequately digest food. My emotions were completely unstable, as was my ability to focus and make decisions. Depression had become my regular daily visitor, or worse yet, an unwelcome, long-term tenant.

When I sat in our nutritionist's office, he asked me what I wanted. I wanted to get rid of my long list of intolerable symptoms. I was tired of being tired. I was sick of being sick. I wanted to be a productive person like I had been before.

Remember that wonderful quote for insanity? "Insanity is

doing what you have always done and expecting a different result."

I laughed when I first heard that. How true this statement is. At first I actually believed that I wouldn't have to change anything to get well. After all, I was a successful person, wasn't I? Why would I have to change anything? What could I possibly be doing wrong?

As the truth of that quote began to sink in, I realized that I was going to have to make some changes. Getting healthy meant I needed to do something different from what I had been doing.

As I shared my story with students, clients, and friends, many people responded with, "How did you really do it? How did you make it work?" I knew *why* I was changing. *Health* was my goal. Sickness and dis-ease were my enemies. Those reasons were meaningful and firmly planted in my heart.

As people listen to or read what I have to share, I encourage them to answer the *why* question for themselves. The response to that question is a personal issue. *You* have to know why *you* want to change.

Successful changers are making a change first of all for themselves.

I have never seen someone make a lasting change in himself or herself only to please someone else. For a change to last, the change had to be important to the person.

Why do you want to change your health or your weight? Are you trying to please someone else? Or is it important to you? If it's not important to *you*, any price will be too expensive for you and you will quit. In your heart you know this is true.

An easy way to think about this *why* question is to ask yourself, "What's in this health change for me? How will I feel after I reach my goal? Is the goal worth the changes that I will have to make?"

In business I learned to answer one question with each client. That question was, "What's in it for me?" An inadequate answer to that question resulted in buyer's remorse and the loss of a sale. After losing one client to buyer's remorse, I became a firm believer in my clients having a clear understanding as to why they were buying a product from me.

When you consider making changes in your life, you are, in effect, buying your desired result. The cost of acquiring that result includes the changes that you will need to make. If you don't want to experience buyer's remorse, know "what is in that result for *you*." Do you really want the result? Are you willing to pay the price to get the result? If you can't answer those questions, buyer's remorse will surely set in.

Successful changers know what's in it for them.

IS THE PROBLEM SIGNIFICANT?

A problem that is significant to you is one that is meaningful to you. I have learned that in order for people to successfully change any area of their life, and especially their health, one of the following two alternatives must be true:

1. The problem must be too costly.
2. The goal must be valuable.

The problem cost or the goal value will dictate the price you are willing to pay. If you realize that neither the cost nor the value is really important to you, you will not change.

In my case my health problems were costing me my life. That was a very expensive set of problems for me and for my family. My depression, weight, mood swings, and other health problems were costing us a great deal of money, time, relationship, and overall satisfaction. The cost was truly considerable!

Cancer patients are totally aware of the cost of their problem. Persons with manic depression are usually aware of their problem. People experiencing a chronic, degenerative dis-ease are usually aware of the costs.

The problem must be costly or the goal must be valuable.

However, not everybody is so aware. If you are unsure of the cost of your health problem, then that cost is probably not very significant to you at this time.

If, however, your problem is significant and costly to you, that very cost can become a prime motivator to you. You pay for your problem on a daily basis, and unless you address it, you will continue to pay for that problem for the remainder of your life.

During your healing process you will probably have the urge to quit many times. When you feel that urge, remind yourself of the cost of that problem. That remembered cost can be an important reminder to you as to why you are changing. During my cleansing time I remember the times I felt like eating a gallon of chocolate-chip ice cream (with a dozen matching cookies, of course). I forced myself to stop and remember being at the hospital. The temptation to eat everything in sight slowly paled in the light of that vivid memory.

Maybe your situation does not appear to be as critical or life-threatening. You are very fortunate. You may have time to prevent such a crisis. It is my prayer that you never, ever have to go through what I went through. And if you are in such a crisis, or close to such a crisis, it is my prayer that you learn from my experience. Come through with flying colors. Begin to experience health as it was meant to be experienced—one day at a time.

IS YOUR GOAL VALUABLE?

Athletes are motivated to reach their goal. They are willing to train, eat right, sleep, exercise—in short, to do whatever is necessary to reach their goal of superior performance.

You may not be an athlete, but your goal may be very valuable to you. Maybe you are tired of being depressed, discontented, and overweight. The depression and weight may not motivate you. Maybe the thought of being joyful, energetic, and slender does motivate you. That is an example of being goal-motivated.

People are motivated differently partly because of their different personality styles. In our family, Forest has amiable, analytic tendencies. He is a nice guy whom everybody immediately trusts and likes. He can research any topic and usually determine the best route to take. He avoids problems. Forest is relaxed and laid-back. If he perceives the cost of a problem to be very high, he will avoid it at any cost. For him, the cost of the problem is his primary motivator.

On the other hand, I have more control tendencies. I am fast-paced, highly energetic, and ready to get a job done immediately. My goals are reached at any cost, whether reasonable or not. I am focused and not too attentive to the details. My goals motivate me. Of course, they do have to be my goals. For me, reaching my goal is my primary motivator.

Early in our marriage, we both "knew" which style was the preferred style. I'm sure you can image what we both "knew."

Over the years we have come to see the benefits of each style. We now know that neither style is better than the other. It is, however, important for us to know which style we are. This is true for you, too. Are you motivated to avoid your problems? Or are you goal-motivated?

Knowing how you are motivated will be invaluable as you answer the *why* question. It can make all the difference in the world when it comes to implementing change strategies. This is true whether the change is for health or some other area of your life.

Know whether you are motivated by problems or goals.

Your primary motivator is your best ally during times of change. When you are unaware of your motivation, you will repeatedly sabotage and frustrate yourself. Your motivator is like free gas. It will fuel you and keep you going when your destination seems far off. Or, it will flame into a hot fire and destroy you.

PAYING THE PRICE

Change is a process of many steps. Habits need to be changed, replaced, or developed. New information needs to assimilated.

Try new food. Learn to do things differently. These steps represent the price you pay to break through health barriers.

Are you beginning to see why it is so important to know how you are motivated? Those steps represent changes that you will need to make on a daily basis. That takes effort. Effort costs you energy. That becomes the price you pay in order to achieve improved health.

You may decide that being healthier isn't worth the hassle. Or you may decide that your problems aren't really that bad after all. If you do, this is probably not the time for you to be trying to change. It's just not worth it to you at this time. That's okay. How much better it is to know that now than after you have spent untold time and money striving to change and failing. Knowing that fact now can keep you out of the yo-yo cycle of failure and allow you to effectively make a change when you are, in fact, ready. You are finally being honest with yourself.

When you do feel like quitting, which you will, remind yourself of why you are changing. That reminder may only keep you going for one more hour. That one hour may be just what you need to stay in the game. This game of life has as many innings as you want to play. There is no one to say, "Strike three, you're out." You just keep on keeping on. Only you decide if you quit.

I remember one time when we were on our cleansing diet. At that time we were eating plain fruits and veggies. One evening Forest and I had an attack of the crunchies. I'm sure you know what that is like. We wanted anything that would go crunch. We imagined potato chips, French fries, cookies, crackers, etc. The sound of crunching was all around us.

Oh, dear! What could we do? My bad memories were vivid. But was that enough to defeat a crunchies attack? I remember saying, "Okay, God, I need some help!"

I remember glancing into one of my many cookbooks. Oh, how inadequate they seemed! Wait! I saw the directions for oven-fried French fries. My creativity began to flow. Regular white potatoes were not allowed yet. We could have yams. Forest and I thinly sliced our yams. We lightly oiled them, sprinkled them with sea salt, and oven-fried them. *Voila!* With our highly awakened imagination, they almost tasted like barbecued potato chips. We ate many yams that evening.

We laugh at the memory of that night. It taught us a very valuable lesson: We could overcome our cravings. Our desire to get healthy was stronger. Creativity helped us win the battle of the crunchies. I was so excited. I had made it through the valley of the crunchies for the first time.

Of course, there have been many battles since then. I have learned, from experience, that I can make it. I occasionally lose a skirmish. However, my motivating desire to be healthy keeps me going. As long as I don't quit, I'm sure to win the war. Losing a skirmish won't cause me to lose the war. Why? Because I simply refuse to quit.

Author Edwin Louis Cole made a great statement in a speech: "You don't drown by falling in the water, you drown by staying there."

My interpretation of that statement is that I won't die from being sick, but I will die if I stay sick. My mistakes here and there won't kill me. Staying in my mistakes (or quitting) can kill me.

HERE COMES THE VELCRO!

The absence of internal motivators during my twenties and early thirties caused me to live a life of Velcro. Prior to knowing about the option of being healthy, I had several ideas as to what I thought I wanted. I wanted to be more successful professionally. Sometimes health seemed like a great goal. Other times, I just didn't care what I did. "Be this, be that" pulled me in many directions. My double-mindedness caused me to operate in a great deal of confusion.

Many opportunities arose to get another college degree. Impulsively, I considered buying exercise machines to improve my health. Hundreds of ads pressured me to buy "the best" diet drink or diet pill. I could never figure out how to spend my money or time because I didn't know what I wanted.

I was vague and double-minded. This double-mindedness was like a big piece of Velcro in my mind. The world exposed my mental Velcro. I encountered all kinds of opportunities. Each one was waiting to attach itself to my big piece of mental Velcro. Guess what? They did. My mind was like a big hodgepodge of Velcro mess. There were colors and shapes stuck all over it. No wonder I didn't know where I was going, and no wonder I wasn't getting anywhere.

Do you ever feel that you just can't seem to get anywhere in the area of health? Do you feel like you are trying to walk in quicksand? Trying too hard causes you to become more stuck. Maybe you are working to get healthy with a lot of misfitting Velcro hanging on you.

What do those misfitting pieces of Velcro look like? One piece could be doing what everybody else says you should do. Thinking that it doesn't really matter what you do today can be a piece of Velcro. There is always tomorrow. Maybe your health problem appears hopeless. It doesn't really matter what you do. This, too, can be a piece of Velcro.

That misfitting Velcro represents our confusion and doubts. Without a clear picture of what we want to achieve, we will allow confusion and doubt to attach themselves to us. As a result, we make our daily health choices based on our shortsighted doubts, fears, and emotions.

When my health crisis hit, I finally realized that how I was living wasn't working. Something had to change. It became apparent that *I* was what had to change. My random, shortsighted choices had produced my health crisis. Not liking that one bit, I decided to change.

I began to map out my plan of action. My plan became defined and valuable to me. Reasonable sacrifices and goals were identified. In time, my picture of health took on clarity, detail, and significance to me.

I denied shortsighted fears, doubts, and emotions (my Velcro) access into my mind. A clear picture of health was glued on my mind and in my heart. Slowly but surely, the sticky old fears, doubts, and confused emotions had no place to stick. I began to get focused on my health.

Determine what it is you want to achieve. Be convinced that

you want your health. If your reasons to get healthy are vague and meaningless, you will be vulnerable to every fear, doubt, and emotion that questions and attacks you. The battle for health is first fought in the mind. You will win or lose your fight for health based on what you allow your mind to attach itself to.

The battle for health is first fought in your mind.

   Clear and meaningful reasons will operate like glue for you. You stick to your goal. You become focused and stronger in your walk of health.

THE HEART OF THE ISSUE:
WHAT IS IMPORTANT TO YOU?

Please do not go any further without spending some quality time answering the following questions. It is very important! My answers have helped move me toward my current level of health. I'm still in process, but I have come so far in such a short period of time.

   Now it's time for you to move on. Take the time to answer these questions honestly. You want to operate with a goal stuck to your mind, not loose Velcro hanging on to every momentary impulse.

1. What does wellness or health mean to you?
2. What health problem(s) do you want to address?
3. *Why* do you want to address this health problem(s)?
4. Is this change important to you?
5. How costly is your health problem?
6. What does your picture of health look like?
7. How valuable is that goal to you?
8. Are you motivated by the cost of your problem or the value of your goal?

   Your past failures in these areas of health can become weights that drag you down. Or, past failures can give you the push you need to move upward and onward out of your pit. Author John Mason says that "the only way to make a comeback is to go on. If the truth were known, 99 percent of success is built on former failure."

An anonymous author wrote this:

> *Success is failure turned inside out,*
> *the silver tint of the clouds of doubt.*
> *You can never tell how close you are.*
> *It may be near when it seems so far.*
> *So stick to the fight when you're hardest hit.*
> *It's when things seem worst that you must not quit.*

You are so close to success! Keep on! You can make it!

CHAPTER SIX

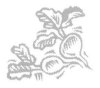

Keep It Simple

If you are like the typical American, you already have a maxed-out schedule. Your calendar is crammed and "free time" is a long-lost luxury. The thought of having the necessary time to make the changes we are talking about may seem laughable to you.

How often do we hear ourselves say, "I just don't have enough time"? Or, "I gotta do this and I gotta do that!" Most people are overcommitted and overwhelmed with their schedules. When something comes along that they really want to do, they have to make sacrifices. Either they can't do the new activity, or they have to sacrifice a commitment. What is the alternative to this madness?

TAKE INVENTORY AND *PRUNE*

Regularly (every three to six months) I take inventory of how I am spending my time. I identify what is most important to me during a season. In nature, we understand the seasons of winter, spring, summer, and fall. Each season has its own purpose for itself and in preparation for the next season. We as people also have seasons.

Our seasons include preparation, family, career, and empty nest or retirement. Obviously this list is not meant to be all-inclusive, nor will it necessarily apply to everyone. It is meant to illustrate the concept of seasonality.

During the preparation season, we are involved as an individual or as a couple in school, education, or on-the-job training. We spend a large amount of our time developing our mental abilities. During the family season, we are usually becoming involved with other people through marriage, childbearing, and child-rearing. This season focuses us on our emotional and social development. During the career season we are focused on developing skills and expertise. We are learning about our calling or purpose for living. This season can help us develop our natural and spiritual gifts for productive use. During the empty-nest or retirement season we are usually readjusting and focusing on outreach to our community and to others. We focus beyond ourselves and share what we have learned with those who are just starting.

Obviously, just as with the natural seasons, our life seasons blend and run into other seasons. Within each season there can be a touch of another season. As we move from one season to another, our time seems to shrink. When we go from just married to married with children, there seems to be no time to do what we used to do. That period is the adjustment period. Taking on more change during an adjustment period is difficult at best and crazy for the average person.

It becomes important to know which season you are in. Are you primarily focused on learning? Maybe you are focused on your marriage and raising your children. Or you're making the big push in your career of developing your calling in life. Maybe the children are gone and you are learning how to reach out to others.

Maybe you are in the midst of several of these seasons. When that is the case, it is critical to become aware of activities that are not necessary to you for that season. For example, if it is spring moving into summer, I should not be focused on my winter wardrobe and when I should wear my warm, woolen sweaters. That is a waste of energy, for it is out of place. However, I might need to have light jackets for cool days and shorts for the warmer days.

So it is with our planning and pruning. Learn to look at each commitment or activity and see if it fits the season you are in. Does that activity or commitment keep you focused, or is it a distraction? Based on your response, start pruning, at least for this season. Just as we set aside clothes after different seasons, so we can set aside activities after a season. Regular pruning of our calendars is critical to having the time to do what is really important to us.

Within seasons we often have several goals at different times. Some are short-term and some are long-term. For example, with our daughter, I have many goals. Some days I have the goal of surviving the day. On other days I am able to focus a little further and work on her character development, which we have as a long-term goal for her. Since I am in both the family and career season, I am continually being challenged to balance them. That was and continues to be a challenge when coupled with working at my health.

When I was in my initial healing process, my main goal was to get healthy. Every commitment and activity was weighed in the light of that goal. If it was helping me get healthier, I kept the activity. If it was not helping me, then it was costing me and I dumped the activity, as least for that time. Even family and career activities were minimal. Learning how to effectively inventory and prune our calendars is an ongoing process. Each time we practice the skill we become better at it.

Take time to inventory and prune your schedule.

When you are working, taking care of a home and family, involved in community activities, *and* you want to get healthier, where do you start? Each piece seems so very important and critical. How could anything be cut? Cutting any piece requires that you set aside an evening or weekend day and allow yourself some uninterrupted time to ponder that question.

You might say, "Right, and where do I get that time?" If, all of a sudden, you were hospitalized with a serious dis-ease, you would have a great deal of time. Don't wait until a crisis like mine or a degenerative dis-ease to take time to address your schedule. Plan to take some time away from your hectic routine. Find the time—your life may depend on it.

When you take that time away from your schedule, identify the season(s) that you are in. Ask yourself what you want to achieve for that season. List the activities you are doing, or would like to do, that help you achieve your goals for that season. From that list, pick the most important two or three. Those activities become your focus for this time period. The other activities are nice, but when your schedule is tight, they become the pieces that send you over the edge into stress and suppression. They also prevent you from having any margin of space.

The key in prioritizing and pruning is to develop a schedule that allows you some margin for the unexpected and for spontaneity. How often have you wanted to take a weekend and go camping or get away as a family? Yet, days turn into months and years and you have not done it. Often that is because every minute within your schedule is filled. Having every minute filled is not an example of a well-ordered schedule. A smooth schedule has room for the unexpected—to help a friend, take a walk, or read to a child. This kind of allowance is necessary to begin to have the freedom to build your health. The lack of it will make health changes too stressful. And once again, the attempts to make health changes will fall by the wayside and be heaped onto the previous failures.

As you prepare to make health changes, take some time and inventory your schedule for the season that you are in. What activity or commitment doesn't fit with that season of your life? Can you reduce or totally eliminate that activity from your schedule? Cut and keep cutting until you have a workable and sensible schedule.

It is okay to take the time to carry out this inventory and pruning process. You don't have to do it in one hour. Don't panic. You have time. Take the time you need to plan your schedule.

Nobody else owns your schedule. You are the person who has to live with it, so keep it as simple as possible.

This leads us into a key principle that will simplify your change process: learning to function in balance.

BE *BALANCED*

How often we hear something new and get excited about it. Within a few days or weeks, our excitement falters and we quit our newest venture. Our "full speed ahead!" screeches to a stand-still. We go from one extreme to the other. No wonder our heads swim from emotional whiplash!

We need to know a few things about balance in order to make effective changes. Don't go from complicated schedules to no schedule at all. Implement a simple schedule. Application needs to be smooth and balanced.

These pointers are not an all-inclusive list. However, they give us some much-needed insight into balance. They come from an excellent tape on time management by Joyce Meyer. Additional information can be obtained by contacting Joyce Meyer at (800)727-9673.

1. New things always come with excitement just because they're new.
2. Excitement will help us get started, but it won't help us finish.
3. Good common sense is usually more helpful than just emotions.
4. People are always looking for "IT."

Being well balanced means to incorporate a combination of things into our lives that will produce fulfillment. There is no one thing that will produce perfect health in you. There is no list of perfect food choices that will work for everybody.

Health, for *you*, is the process of finding that combination of things that work just for you. It takes time to become healthy, in a balanced manner. Each person will need to do something just a little differently than the next person. You and your body are unique. So your healing process is unique to you.

We all love anything new. There is something so exciting about getting something new, starting something new, or being somewhere new. Newness, by itself, is exciting. We have lots of energy when we are excited. We feel like we could run miles and conquer the world when we are excited.

Many people make hasty decisions during this rush of adrenaline. The next morning, when their adrenaline high is gone, they wonder why they ever made such a crazy commitment or decision. Sound familiar? Excitement is very fickle; it can get you into many things but it never sticks around to help you finish.

Be balanced in your changes— don't overreact!

Being well balanced means using common sense, not just emotions, to make commitments and decisions. Along with common sense, use some wisdom. Wisdom helps you to know how to best apply knowledge in a way that will work for you at this time. Rules and formulas will not bring balance to our lives, but common sense will.

As you read about the suggested food choices in the "Food for the Body" chapters, remember to keep it simple. Sleep on your decisions. Ask yourself, "Do I have the time to make this change now?" Take each change one step at a time. Apply your changes with common sense. I can guarantee that you will need to customize most suggestions in order for them to work for you. Those choices will take effort and energy to carry out. As you apply each new choice, do it with balance.

The result of imbalance is stress and sickness. Many people have ignored the health consequences of their fast-paced, stress-driven lives. They inhale food that is lacking nutrition, while they consume chemically laden beverages instead of pure water. Magical drinks or pills are swallowed to melt away their flab. Pills are popped to suppress their symptoms of dis-ease. They end up totally stressed and sick.

People often go from one extreme to another. From poor

health habits, they overreact by trying every available health fad. When nothing seems to work, they wonder why they feel like such a total failure. Self-pity raises its ugly head. Our bodies are amazingly versatile. However, even that versatility reaches a point of no return. Whizzing from one extreme to another is the ultimate definition of imbalance.

Effective change requires balance. Take one step at a time. When you start to feel overwhelmed, back off. Feeling overwhelmed comes from trying to do much at once. Look and identify where you are trying to do too much. Pick one thing and do it. Wait until you're ready to add something else. Take a deep breath and remind yourself to keep it simple.

As I learned to keep things simple, I became much more aware of my time. I finally acknowledged and accepted a golden rule of time: There are only twenty-four hours in a day. No matter how successful, strong-willed, or intelligent I may be, I can't change that golden rule. I may become more efficient in my use of time, but the number of hours in my day will never change.

The variable in time management is never the amount of time, it is our use of that time. Have you heard yourself say, "I don't have time to do this or that"? Guess what? The amount of time you have is never going to change. It is what you do within that twenty-four hours a day and seven days a week that can change. Learning to use our time wisely and simply leads us to effective time management.

> *Healthier people know there are only twenty-four hours in a day.*

Imbalanced people are driven by the loud voice of "should." How many times have we said, "I should eat better food" or "I should exercise" or "I should slow down"? Have you ever noticed that you rarely get around to doing the "shoulds" in your life? Have you ever wondered why? It's simple; shoulds aren't really important to us. Shoulds are also from the parental voice in us— one we naturally rebel against. We do what we want to do. We ignore the shoulds.

If your health is in the realm of a "should" instead of a "want to," you are setting yourself up for failure. Answer the *why* questions found in chapter 5. You will move your health into the realm of "want to" and out of the losing battleground of "should." Leave the shoulds behind. You will be doing more of what you want to do.

MAKE ONE CHANGE AT A TIME

A simple key to remember during your healing process is to choose one area of change at a time. You don't have to carry out all of the possible changes at once. It is humanly impossible to simultaneously do all that is available to do to get healthy. Why? Because you are a human being, with a finite ability to adjust to change.

Remember the family that decided to omit sugar from their diet? They worked on that one area for almost twelve months. Removing sugar seemed simple. They were excited to begin their changes. Excitement waned as they began to read labels. Sugar, or one of its aliases, was in nearly everything they ate. A simple decision took nearly a year to implement. The excitement disappeared long before the end of that year.

Change one thing at a time.

I remember the first time I went to a health-food store to buy a few items. A five-minute job, or so I thought, ended up taking almost an hour. I didn't know my way around the store. Many vegetables were unfamiliar to me. It was embarrassing to ask a produce clerk to identify my vegetables for me. I felt so stupid.

If you have children, you can probably remember when they first began to learn how to walk. First, they learned to stand up and pull themselves up. Over and over they practiced. Next came the balancing act. Slowly they took their first step, and immediately fell. We applauded their every practice session. They would get back up and try again.

Children are a wonderful example of simplicity. They focus

Keep It Simple

on one thing and practice it repeatedly. Today, most of us find walking to be so simple we rarely think about it. Why? Because we practiced it every day until we could do it simply and easily. We kept it simple. We mastered the skill.

Replace dis-ease running with health walking.

You are learning to walk in the area of health. Your walking may feel much slower than your old style of running. That is okay. Walking is supposed to be slower than running. It is always better to walk with health than to run with dis-ease.

We often feel dumb when we are slow at something. Did you know that is a definition of simple? A "simple" person can be perceived as slow, common, or perhaps even foolish. I would be rather be simply healthy than intelligently dis-eased.

CHANGE FEELS AWKWARD!

Usually it is pride that causes us to not want to appear foolish to others. My goodness, what will other people think? Our imaginations run wild with the possibilities of other people's perceptions of us. Vain imaginations can hold us hostage to undesirable situations.

Memories of my gym-joining days came flooding back. Each time I decided to join, I had the very best of intentions. But the second I walked into that kingdom of beautifully proportioned, slender bodies, I questioned every part of that well-conceived decision. What would all of those slender people think of my not-so-slender body? My sense of inadequacy was extreme, to say the least. My body did not move like my teacher's body. Her movements and my movements had very little in common. I felt so awkward! Although I was just starting to exercise, I compared myself to my teacher.

When we begin to learn something, we have to allow ourselves time to learn. Learning is a process, and feeling inadequate and awkward is part of that process. We are not a failure because we feel inadequate and awkward. These sensations are very normal. We will not immediately be like our teachers. Our teachers invested time and much effort to develop their skills and expertise.

Feeling awkward is feeling clumsy, embarrassed, or uncomfortable. Feeling uncomfortable is in direct contradiction to the excitement we first feel when we start something new. Because of that emotional conflict, many people stop at that awkward stage. When they stop, they are choosing to stay stuck in their yo-yo cycle of start-stop, start-stop. Give yourself time to become comfortable in your new choices.

> *It's normal to feel awkward and inadequate when learning a new skill.*

Success includes the awkward and inadequacy phase. We have all experienced going through the awkwardness of learning to walk. Most of us have made it through the awkwardness of puberty.

If we want to become healthy, we have to allow ourselves the freedom to feel awkward. We are learning new skills. It will take some time before those new skills feel comfortable. That is normal. If you don't feel awkward at all, you probably aren't experiencing any real change.

As we summarize keeping it simple, consider the following quotation from an anonymous author:

Approach it simply in your thinking, and it won't be complicated in your doing!

When you start to feel overwhelmed, stop. Slow down and identify what really needs to be done, one simple step at a time. Take the time to think it through. Let each step be simple. Don't make everything so complicated.

As you work on simplifying your lifestyle, you will want to begin to seek out a source of encouragement. Encouragement is the act of giving courage, hope, or confidence to a person. It is supportive and uplifting. During change, encouragement is our lifeline. It keeps us going when we don't always want to. Courage grows, hope mounts, and confidence increases with encouragement.

Living without encouragement is like living without light or sunshine. The darkness overwhelms us. Constant darkness stunts growth. Plants wither and die when left in the dark. People die when exposed to a steady diet of discouragement.

Encouragement notes progress. Discouragement sees only failures and unfinished activities. Encouragers spotlight your progress during the process of change. Discouraging people point out your failures and deficiencies. Be choosy.

Be aware of your progress. Progress, by its very definition, means "forward movement, a development or an improvement." Problems can overwhelm us and cause us to feel sorry for ourselves, which quickly stops our progress.

> *Choose encouragers and reject discouraging people.*

STOP CRITICIZING AND START ENCOURAGING!

Having had a perfectionistic nature, I often belittled my progress. I still catch this trait in my relationship with our daughter. She brings her papers home from school. Immediately, my eyes fly to the red marks. I don't see a paper with forty-eight right answers. I see a paper with two wrong answers. It is so easy to notice the two wrong answers and ignore the forty-eight right ones. Our basic human nature gravitates toward the negative. Seeing the positive is a learned trait.

We do the same thing to ourselves. We criticize ourselves, while we ignore our progress. It is important to learn to acknowledge our progress. Each step of progress represents much work. Congratulate yourself on your progress! Stop criticizing yourself for not being perfect. You will never be perfect or perfectly healthy. *Remember*: Health is a process, not a destination in your life.

We encourage our daughter by acknowledging her appropriate

choices. As she feels our love and support, her behavior improves at home and school. Sometimes her behavior slips. After investigating the situation, I often find that my interaction with her had slipped. I find myself saying, "Do this!" "Why did you do that?" "Why did you miss that?" "Don't you ever listen?" That form of communication needs revision. Her behavior quickly improves with better communication from me.

The old adage "Honey catches more flies than vinegar" is true. We see more positive results when we use encouraging words. Nagging, critical words are sour. This is especially true in the area of food. Constantly nagging someone about food is a nightmare for everybody. Be positive in your discussion of food.

Barking commands of "Don't eat that!" "Go exercise, now!" "Why did you eat that?" causes discouragement and failure. Learn to replace negative words with encouraging words. Acknowledge improvement and enjoy its benefits. Encouraging progress won't stop development. It will cause development to happen more smoothly and quickly.

LIFE IS A PROCESS, NOT JUST A SERIES OF GOALS

Acknowledging progress has helped me understand that life is a process. I used to see life as a goal or event. One day I would *arrive* and not have any more problems. That is a misconception and a delusion. So much life is missed waiting for the arrival of events.

How many of us miss out on life because we wait for results or goals? Our lives become one scheduled event after another. We forget to smell the roses along the way.

Savor each moment of your life.

Life is a combination of steps, events, and goals. It takes time. I am learning to enjoy the process. As a result, I am enjoying my life as I have never enjoyed it before.

Focusing on results alone can cause us to miss much fun. I remember planning for Christmas. I figured out the perfect gift for each person. Each perfect gift required hours and hours of work. I scrambled and rushed to get everything done "on schedule." When Christmas rolled around, the "event" was over in one hour. What a letdown! What had happened to all of the fun? Ignoring the process, I had strived for the goal and missed the fun of the moment.

Enjoy yourself as you go through your changes. Don't wait until you are perfectly healthy to decide to enjoy yourself. Have fun now! Today is part of your life. Don't miss it. A perfect tomorrow never comes. Enjoy today for all it is worth.

One of my friends decided to make some significant changes in her diet. She called and asked if I would be willing to be one of her supporters. I said yes. She called frequently, ready to quit.

As she talked, her wavering emotions spoke loudly. They ricocheted from sentence to sentence. She was unsure of everything. I encouraged her to stop and look at her progress. At first, I reminded her that she had made it one week. Then I reminded her of a month's worth of progress. Soon I was reminding her that she had steadily improved her health for eleven months.

Often during my healing process, my emotions wavered and I, too, felt like quitting. Hopelessness overwhelmed me. I learned to make it five minutes at a time. Handling five more minutes seemed possible. The thought of an hour or a day was too much. I learned to offer my friends the same encouragement.

Now we laugh at the hundreds of five-more-minutes through which we have come. We were encouraged and comforted so often by those words. Five more minutes helped put our frustrations and problems in perspective. We silence our wavering emotions for some needed quiet. Soon, we can think clearly and come to our own conclusion. Yes, we can make it five more minutes!

"You can make it five more minutes."

HAVE FUN!

Being a serious person, I have had to learn to have fun and to laugh. It is okay to laugh at myself and have a sense of humor.

Forest has a wonderfully unique sense of humor. Our daughter has a unique variation of her dad's humor. Being in a family with them has destined me to laughter. I must laugh or cry in frustration at their humor.

Most healthy people have learned to laugh and keep things in perspective. They don't take themselves too seriously. They acknowledge their blessings.

It's not always easy to see the humor in a current situation. This is especially true if the situation is

Laughter really is good medicine!

painful or difficult. However, we can learn to look for the humor. When I find myself getting too serious, I try to remember some of our many humorous moments. Believe me, there are plenty of those moments! Laughter allows me to relax and enjoy life more than ever before.

As I tell my story in seminars, I share the humor in it. Otherwise, people become depressed. People love entertainment, and laughter is a great source of entertainment.

Retelling my suicide story got boring and morbid. One day I remembered a funny scene from that incident. Remember the dramatic suicide scenes in the movies? The hero or heroine pours a bottle of pills into his or her cupped hands. Dramatically this person throws back his or her head and swallows all of the pills. My memory was different from that image. Only one pill at a time can go down my narrow throat. So, instead of dramatically swallowing a handful of pills, I took each pill, one at a time.

That memory has allowed me to tell my story with humor. As a result, I have a different perspective of myself. Although my message is serious, I don't need to be serious all of the time. I lighten up. The audience lightens up and we all enjoy ourselves.

That same technique works during stressful changes. Learn to see the humor in the moment. Never laugh at the expense of another person. Making fun of someone else will only cause pain. Learn to take things and people less seriously. Don't overreact. Health is a serious issue. However, you don't have to live seriously to become healthy.

FIND SUPPORTIVE PEOPLE

As I rebuilt my health, I surrounded myself with supportive people. Not everybody was supportive of my decision to get healthy. That was an amazing fact to me.

I discovered that some people feel better when we have problems. Our problems give them the excuse they need to stay in their own problem. These people discourage us to the point of quitting. They criticize us and are a negative influence. All of our best intentions are sabotaged by their negativity. I removed those people from my life.

As I got stronger, I knew I could change that choice, but living without negative people is an addictive habit. Soon, I didn't miss negative people at all. I like having positive, encouraging friends. Today, I reduce the time I spend with negative, critical people.

We become like the people with whom we associate. During a time of healing, it is very important to surround yourself with healthy people. These people need to be as physically, emotionally, and mentally healthy as possible. You want to be around people who encourage you in getting healthy. Do not be around people who prefer to see you keep your problems.

Our attitudes, thoughts, and friends operate like a construction plumb line. Using a plumb line causes the construction of a building to stay straight. A straight building is less likely to topple during a storm. A builder follows the plumb line. When he sees that he is leaning too far to the right, he adjusts and moves to the left.

Discouraging attitudes, thoughts, and friends will kill us. They pull us toward hopelessness and failure. They remind us of what we haven't done. On the other hand, selecting encouraging attitudes, thoughts, and friends can help us as we construct our health. When we're discouraged, they support us with hope and confidence. They will remind us that we can make it, if only five minutes at a time.

Part Three
Food for the Body

CHAPTER SEVEN

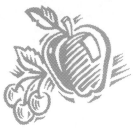

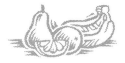

Where Do I Start?

D r. C. Everett Koop published a report on nutrition and health in October 1988. He left no doubt about the urgent need to alter our eating habits to stem the growth of disease that affects our population. Presently in the United States, 2.1 million people die annually from all causes of death. Diet plays a role in 68 percent of these deaths. If you remove suicide and unintentional injuries such as auto accidents from the list of causes, *the number of deaths to which diet is a factor is a whopping 80 percent.*[1]

What we eat is critical to our total health. We all know that, but we seem to overlook it when we make our daily food choices. Using food to bring health is not a new idea. Hippocrates, author of the Hippocratic oath, said, "Let food be thy medicine."

Another person who furthered the medicinal value of food was Victor Rocine. He analyzed and measured the effect of chemical elements in our many common foods. Rocine was very knowledgeable about the impact food played on the body. His works were summarized in the following quotation:

If we eat wrongly,
No doctor can cure us;

If we eat rightly,
No doctor is needed.

Let's look at a more contemporary person. Dr. Norman Walker, health practitioner for over 80 years, died at the age of 109. His beliefs and practices produced a life of tremendous vitality and health. In his book, *Diet and Salad*, he gave an excellent analogy of the impact of food on the body. An individual of 40 years, eating three meals a day, will have consumed more than 40,000 meals to date. For the average person, most of that food has been cooked, canned, or processed.

The result of more than 40,000 meals, composed mostly of dead food (or inorganic chemical elements) have passed through this system during that time. *It is impossible to regenerate organic cells in a human body with inorganic (or dead) matter.* These meals serve the purpose of sustaining life. Hardly any nourishment was eaten to regenerate the cells and tissues of the body.[2]

Another contemporary supporter of preventive health is John A. McDougall, M.D. In his book, *McDougall's Medicine: A Challenging Second Opinion*, he states:

The normal state of the body is health not illness. The body has an innate ability to heal and maintain health once the factors causing the disease are removed. Since dietary and lifestyle factors cause most chronic disease, the key to regaining health is to correct these factors. *Without a strong body, with the capacity to mend itself, no amount of medication will regain health.*[3]

We know food is critical to health. Most of us want more than sickness, dis-ease, or mere existence. An abundant life is our goal. We don't want to live at a doctor's office or in the hospital. If we agree to this goal, where do we start?

START SLOWLY

In as simple terms as possible, I recommend that you move from white, dead, packaged foods to whole, colorful, varied, alive foods. The closer you are to a white (white flour, sugar, rice, etc.) packaged diet, the unhealthier you are. The more colorful (fresh fruits and vegetables, etc.) and natural (for example, whole grains) your diet, the healthier you are. That is a simple scale to understand. Moving from the white end to the colorful end is a process. You decide how quickly and thoroughly you want to move.

Whatever approach you take, it is usually best to move slowly. Changing your customary eating habits completely and suddenly can cause more temporary discomfort than you would like. This discomfort is commonly called a healing crisis. Often it is avoidable by using a balanced, sensible approach to dietary changes.

Healing-crisis symptoms occur because the body is ridding itself of toxic substances. These substances are ejected out of the tissues and into the body's system. While the toxins are in the body system, before elimination, the body is temporarily more toxic.

A brief composite of sample cleanses is in appendix A of this book (see page 175). Whether you choose to do a cleanse or not, these twenty-five suggested starting places will be helpful. Seventeen appear in this chapter. Eight more are in chapter 8.

WHERE CAN I START?

In the following information, I will share some changes our family made as we learned how to make smart food choices. These suggestions are not an all-inclusive list but a place to start. Everybody can find something in this list that will work for them, wherever they are.

As we discussed in the "Food for Thought" chapters, health is a process. The more you learn about health, the more you realize you don't know. Our body has the amazing ability to adapt to whatever we do. The more health principles I learn and apply, the better my body feels.

Read these suggestions. Discuss them with your family. It is okay to choose just one suggestion to apply for now. Obviously, doing all of the suggestions produces more health. However, usually that is not a balanced, sensible approach.

With the help of a qualified health-care practitioner, you can find the best selection and order of suggestions for you. Each step brings you closer to your desired health. Each subsequent step becomes a little easier than the previous step. We thoroughly enjoy the food we now eat and have no desire to revert to our old eating habits. The return has far outweighed the cost and inconvenience of our change process.

Release your creativity as you consider each suggestion. I will offer several original implementation ideas that have worked for us. However, don't let those ideas limit you. Customize your application. The better the changes work for you, the longer the changes will last.

One—Tour a Health-Food Store
Have you ever been in a health-food store? If not, I highly encourage you to visit one. You may be asking, "What exactly is health food, anyway?" Health food includes fresh produce (organic when possible), whole grains and beans, and packaged food made without additives and chemicals. It could also include dairy products produced without growth hormones or other chemicals, as well as meat, poultry, and fish raised without hormones and chemicals. Health food can be some of the tastiest food available. As you learn the quality brands (see appendix C, page 204), you will wonder why you didn't start purchasing "health food" sooner.

Health-food stores have an atmosphere totally different from today's supermarket. I have been in health-food stores throughout the country. Shopping in them is a welcome change from large supermarkets. Why? Their smaller size promotes a calmer atmosphere. The staff is friendly and approachable. They are informative and extremely knowledgeable about the different departments.

I remember when Forest and I first started eating healthier. At that point our financial situation was as bad as my health condition. Altalta's, our local health-food store, had wonderful complimentary cooking classes. The class became our "free" date for the evening. After the samples (our dinner), we toured the store aisles. A great deal about food was learned during those dates. What a great time we had! Since then we have become true supporters of our health-food stores.

You may not have the privilege of living in a community with a health-food store. Although this is becoming less of a problem, it may be a problem for you. If it is, become aware of mail-order resources. Appendix B lists mail-order options.

Health food can also be purchased from some wholesalers through food cooperatives (co-ops). Sources of wholesalers throughout the country can also be found in appendix B.

Two—Keep a Food Diary

Today, few people keep a diary or journal. Even fewer keep track of their finances beyond their checkbook. As a result, we have forgotten the role a diary can play.

A diary is a written record of our experiences in a given area. A food diary records the food we eat. Because food is such a subtle habit, many of us are unaware of the type and quantity of food we eat.

Food diaries were used by my nutritionist to track low-grade food allergies. I kept track of the food eaten, the time it was eaten, and my general reactions. My food diary pinpointed food sensitivities, emotional eating patterns, and food repetitions.

It is so easy to eat the same thing on a repetitious basis without realizing it. Food repetition is a common cause of many food allergies. Detecting emotional eating patterns helped me break the habits more easily. I learned to provide alternate foods during emotional lows.

As with all of these suggestions, a food diary is your choice. However, your actual food intake might surprise you. A food diary will give you accurate information on your daily food intake. Knowing where you are is a prerequisite to get to a new place.

Three—Read Labels

This sounds obvious. However, many people today are unaware of the contents of food, other than its fat content. Fat content is important and we will discuss it later. Equally important is chemical content. Replacing high-fat foods with chemicals (that is, preservatives or additives), sugar, fillers, or food coloring is not a wise choice. That is merely replacing one enemy with another.

Let's take a look at a couple of labels and walk through this process. These foods were selected only because they have relatively few ingredients in their list. Many ingredient labels are quite long.

The first product is Pop-Tarts. A cherry Pop-Tart label lists the following:

▶ cherry filling (corn syrup)—a sugar
▶ dextrose—a sugar
▶ cherries—a food item
▶ crackermeal—a food item
▶ wheat starch—a food filler
▶ apples—a food item
▶ partially hydrogenated soybean oil—a poor-quality fat
▶ citric acid—an additive
▶ xanthan gum—a food thickener
▶ red #40—a food coloring, a chemical
▶ natural flavoring—this can be anything
▶ blue #1—food coloring, a chemical
▶ enriched wheat flour—this means enriched white flour that acts like sugar in the body
▶ partially hydrogenated soybean oil—a poor-quality fat
▶ corn syrup—a sugar
▶ sugar—a sugar
▶ whey—a dairy byproduct
▶ baking powder—a food item
▶ baking soda—a food item

Of the nineteen ingredients in this product, only five are food items. Those five appear on the list lower than two sugar items, which means there is more sugar than cherries, cracker-meal, or apples. The other two food items are baking powder and baking soda.

How about a staple like peanut butter? A well-known brand's label has the following ingredients:

► roasted peanuts—a food item
► sugar—a sugar
► partially hydrogenated vegetable oil—a poor-quality fat
► salt—salt, high in sodium

In contrast, another brand of "health" peanut butter (by Roaster Fresh) has the following ingredient listed on its labels:

► peanuts—a food item

Nothing but peanuts is used to make this peanut butter. A real difference can be found among products. This is why we included a list of preferred brands in appendix C. Begin to look at food labels. Start by looking at the food in your pantry. Are the ingredients building, neutral to, or tearing down your health? You are eating those ingredients. Nobody makes the buying decisions for your food but you.

I have two simple rules of thumb for labels. First, if I can't say or spell the ingredients, I don't buy the item. Second, if I couldn't create a recipe with the ingredients, I don't buy the product.

I buy only those products made from food. Most packaged food is made of chemicals and other artificial ingredients. They do not produce health. I want my money to buy food, not chemicals.

A real misnomer on labels is the word *natural. Natural* can mean anything. Poison can be 100-percent natural. Get beyond the marketing buzzwords found on labels. Go to the small print. The small print on a label is the ingredient list. The ingredients are what you are buying.

Business will try to sell you packaging, slogans, ads, and

other allurements. You may pay for them, but you don't eat them. The packaging may be convenient, which is fine. However, you eat the contents. Learn to check out what you are buying.

As you practice reading labels, you will begin to note manufacturers that abide by high-quality standards. I now buy from certain vendors regularly. Their attention to quality has made me a loyal customer.

In all of my cookbooks I give a list of preferred vendors and brands by food type. Why? I am not compensated by any of these vendors. I know what it is like to stand in an aisle without the signposts of General Foods and Kraft to guide me. Which new brand do I buy? The decision process can be overwhelming.

When switching to health food, it is good to know where to start. A list of preferred brands represents a good starting place. My selection criteria included taste, quality of ingredients, price, and availability. A copy of that list can be found in appendix C.

Four—Eat More Vegetables
Most of us know we need to eat vegetables. Under our breaths, we say "YUK!" Vegetables are not sweet, salty, or fatty. They have no taste at all! Our taste buds and minds reject veggies.

People who eat large quantities of processed food, from packaged food to fast food, have desensitized taste buds. The sense of taste can be compared to drug and alcohol addictions. The more addicted a person is to cocaine, the more cocaine is needed to produce a high. Taste buds are similar. Chemically laden foods desensitize our taste buds. The more we eat of this type of food, the more we want it. We need more of it to awaken our sense of taste.

It takes approximately two weeks of eating clean foods for the taste buds to be cleansed. Clean food is live food, or food without chemicals and added processing. Once the taste buds are clean, simple foods and beverages have flavor. Before you discount vegetables, cleanse your taste buds.

You might be saying, "I still don't like vegetables!" I have found a couple of ways to address this issue for myself. When I first knew that I needed to eat salads, I had the same response:

"I hate salads!" However, I knew that green stuff was good for me. So I found a few dressings (as low in fat as possible) and covered my salad with dressing. I know that lots of dressing is not particularly healthy. But over time (several years) I found that I could reduce the quantity of dressing and eat more salad. I can now eat a normal salad with a small amount of dressing.

I have taken a different approach with beets. I know that beets are one of the best vegetables for the liver. That knowledge did not erase the fact that I didn't like the flavor or the texture of beets. However, the taste did not make me gag. So, I found that I could "tune out" or ignore the food and just eat it. I don't eat them often, but I have learned to tolerate that vegetable. When I'm not up to ignoring the taste, I just double the quantity of my dark green leafy vegetables.

Another approach I have used is with wheat-grass juice, considered by many health-food experts to be one of the most perfect foods available. It is merely wheat grass (green grass, before it heads out into wheat shafts) that is run through a special juicer to extract the green juice. It is very rich in chlorophyll and minerals. With my first taste of wheat grass, I felt like I had died and *not* gone to heaven. It was awful! Knowing it was so nutritious, I occasionally looked for new ways to try this drink. I finally found a palatable way. To one ounce of wheat-grass juice, I add eight ounces of fresh apple juice and a splash of fresh lime juice, to taste. This combination is actually not bad. I can now tolerate wheat-grass juice.

Of course, there may be a few vegetables for which none of these approaches work for you. However, with the wide variety of vegetables, there will be many vegetables that will help you get your basic nutrition. Every so often, give that difficult vegetable a try. If you are like me, you will hate to be beaten by a mere vegetable. I put my creativity to work and continue to look for ways to make the difficult vegetables more palatable for me and my family.

Now that we know vegetables can have flavor, which ones do we eat? Another simple rule of thumb applies. The more intense the color of the vegetable, the higher the nutrient level.

For example, yams have more nutrients than white potatoes.

The one vegetable that is close to worthless is iceberg lettuce. Recently a student shared her observations on iceberg lettuce. She was learning to feed her family more veggies. During each trip to the produce section, she reviewed the nutritional information found on cards above the individual items. On the iceberg lettuce card, the nutritional analysis said: "Good for tacos." No other nutritional benefit was listed on the card.

Replace iceberg with quality green leaf lettuce. Leaf lettuce is much more attractive. As your eyes become adjusted to leaf lettuce, you will wonder how anybody could eat pale, tasteless iceberg.

Maybe you think veggies are limited to peas, corn, carrots, and potatoes. Vegetables are far more varied than that. The following list contains some available vegetables.

artichokes	mustard greens
asparagus	okra
bamboo shoots	onions
beets	parsley
broccoli	potatoes
Brussels sprouts	pumpkin
cabbage	radishes
carrots	rutabagas
cauliflower	scallions
celery	shallots
chili peppers	sorrel
corn	spinach
cucumbers	sprouts
eggplant	squashes
escarole	sweet potatoes
garlic	Swiss chard
gingerroot	tomatoes
kale	turnips
leeks	watercress
lettuce	yams
mushrooms	zucchini

That list may overwhelm you. What have we learned to do with things that overwhelm? We stop and take one step at a time. That list is your smorgasbord, not your grocery list. You get to choose from that list.

I recommend trying one new vegetable a week. That is a simple step to apply. Vegetables can be eaten raw, baked, steamed, or stir-fried. They can be placed in soups, in casseroles, or on pizzas. Knowing a variety of cooking methods increases your enjoyment of vegetables. When in doubt as to the best form of preparation, refer to a good health cookbook (see appendix H, page 229, for a list of recommended cookbooks), or ask your market's produce staff.

Try adding a different raw vegetable to your salad. Using the vegetable in small amounts can help the trial periods go more easily. Vary the colors of vegetables that you eat. Eating a full range of colors improves the probability that you are getting a full range of vitamins and minerals.

Eat six half-cup servings of fruits and vegetables each day. Eat as much variety in your veggies as possible. That means that vegetables, not meat, become your main food group. Build your meals around vegetables. We will discuss this more in our chapter on meal planning.

Within the vegetable family, sweet potatoes and yams are considered the most nutritious. They are the highest-ranked vegetables in the percentage of vitamins A and C, calcium, iron, and copper. Carrots rank second, with collard greens, red peppers, kale, dandelion greens, spinach, and broccoli following closely.

Tomatoes, although a fruit, are often eaten with vegetables. Like citrus fruits, they are highly acidic. As a part of the nightshade family, they purportedly promote arthritis. If the tomato seeds are green, the tomato is neither ripe nor edible. The yellow variety is the best because it is a nonacid fruit.

Five—Eat More Fruits

Since fruits are naturally sweeter than vegetables, most people find fruit easier to eat. As a rule of thumb, vegetables are a better source of minerals and fruits are a better source of vitamins. This is only true when fruits have had the necessary time to ripen and fully develop before being picked.

Unlike vegetables, fruits ripen in the sun. That ripening process affects the fruit's sweetness and flavor. The riper the fruit, the better it is for you. Dried fruit, eaten sparingly, is acceptable. The drying process concentrates the fruit sugar.

As with vegetables, fruits should be eaten seasonally. Eating seasonally automatically brings variety to our diet. A seasonal food chart can be found in appendix D, page 216.

What are our fruit options besides apples, bananas, and oranges? Here is a list of fruits.

apples	lemons
apricots	limes
bananas	mangoes
blackberries	nectarines
blueberries	oranges
boysenberries	papayas
cantaloupe	peaches
casaba	pears
cherries	pineapple
cranberries	plantains
currants	plums
dates	pomegranates
figs	prunes
grapefruit	raisins
grapes	raspberries
guava	strawberries
honeydew melon	tangelos
kiwi	tangerines
kumquats	watermelon

The best way to eat fruit is raw and ripe. Citrus fruit can affect the body's acidity. Therefore, eat citrus fruits in small quantities.

Six—Eat Food That Has Been Cleaned

Clean produce is essential. I believe that the best form of produce is organic. Although there is no documented scientific evidence to prove that statement, I believe common sense can. The fewer chemicals, fertilizers, and pesticides used to grow produce, the cleaner the produce. That is a logical conclusion to me. As much as availability and budget allow, we buy organic produce. Your body will appreciate the difference found in organic produce. Eventually, your taste buds will, too.

When organic produce is not available, food cleansing becomes even more critical. Merely washing fruits and vegetables, organic or not, with water is not enough. There are several commercial produce washes available.

My favorite produce wash is also very inexpensive. I place a few drops of Shaklee's Basic H (Amway LOC can also be used) in a sink of water and let the produce soak for ten to thirty minutes. Then I place the washed produce into a dish drainer to drain.

To purchase a Shaklee or Amway product, contact a local sales rep. You can usually find a list of names in the white business pages of your local phone book. Shaklee and Amway referrals can be obtained by contacting their headquarters at (800)SHAKLEE and (800)544-7167, respectively. A quart of either product costs under ten dollars and will last for a long time. Be sure to ask the rep how to use the product for other forms of cleaning. Both products are excellent general, nontoxic household cleaners.

Using Basic H or LOC with water works on all produce from lettuce to potatoes. It does not work well with mushrooms. All of our produce hits the sink before it hits our mouth. The amount of dirt and grit left at the bottom of a sink from a produce wash will amaze you. You were ingesting that grit before.

Seven—Store Foods Correctly to Prevent Spoilage

Processed food has a questionable benefit over health food. It has a longer shelf life. The reason the shelf life is so long is because the food is dead. Although it can last forever on the shelf, dead food does little, if any, work in your body.

Eating live, healthy food requires different food-storage techniques. Store all cold processed oils (discussed under point eleven) in your refrigerator to prevent rancidity. The only exception to this rule is olive oil, which can be kept at room temperature.

Store whole grains in airtight containers. A bay leaf or stick of peppermint gum can be used to keep out bugs. The bakery department in many grocery stores will provide empty five-gallon frosting buckets at minimal or no charge. These buckets work well for whole grains.

Store fresh whole-grain flours in the freezer or refrigerator. This prevents the natural oils found in the flour from going rancid. Fresh whole-grain flours have a naturally sweet taste. The older the flour, the less sweet it is.

Refrigerating nuts prevents rancidity and also helps protect the nuts' natural moisture content.

Purchase dry herbs and spices in small quantities and store in airtight containers. Health-food stores are a great source for herbs, as the bulk pricing makes them much cheaper than in a supermarket. These herbs are also fresher and more flavorful. Usually, health-food-store herbs have had fewer chemical processes.

Fresh herbs can be stored in the refrigerator for a time. When they start to droop, they can be frozen or dried. Fresh herbs are more nutritious than dried herbs. They also have more flavor. Fresh herbs can be easily grown in a pot in a kitchen window, on a patio, or in a garden. They are very hardy and grow like weeds. If possible, select organic seeds.

Eight—Eat Food in the Healthiest Form Possible
The closer food is to its raw form, the better. Raw foods contain enzymes. Enzymes are the source of energy from which the body functions. When food provides the enzymes, the body does not have to produce them. This reduces the work performed by the liver.

Cooking at high temperatures kills enzymes. Most processed foods have small amounts of enzymes. Most people do not want to go to a totally raw diet. However, the amount of raw food eaten is directly linked to frequency and seriousness of dis-ease. Eat a raw salad daily. If possible, eat raw veggies for snacks. The more raw fruits and veggies consumed, especially veggies, the better off you are.

While in Dallas, Texas, doing a book signing at a Whole Foods Market, I learned more about organic food. The following points summarize this information.

▶ Since the 1940s crop losses inflicted by insect pests have nearly doubled from 7 percent to 13 percent, despite a tenfold increase in insecticide use.

▶ There are an estimated 45,000 human acute poisonings from pesticides each year, about 3,000 of which are serious enough to hospitalize the patient. This figure does not include the potential problems with cancer that may come later.

▶ Many imported fruits and vegetables, primarily from Latin America, are exposed to heavy doses of pesticides now banned in the United States. One of the most-sprayed fruits are grapes from Chile.

▶ Over 50 percent of imported apples, bell peppers, cabbage, carrots, cantaloupe, celery, cherries, cucumbers, grapefruit, lettuce, peaches, strawberries, and tomatoes analyzed by the Food and Drug Administration (FDA) contained pesticide residues. Of these, imported bell peppers, cantaloupe, cucumbers, strawberries, and tomatoes had especially high incidence (over 70 percent pesticide residues).

▶ Certain produce is more likely to contain pesticides than others. Strawberries top the list, followed by peaches, celery, cherries, cucumbers, bell peppers, and tomatoes.

▶ More pesticide residues are detected in strawberries than any other fruit.

▶ Celery contains more pesticide residues than any other vegetable.

▶ According to the Department of Agriculture, nearly

half the total quantity of pesticides applied in the nation are used in corn production.

Obviously, food that contains fewer chemicals is better. The above information can help you decide which produce to buy commercially and which to buy organic. If organic produce is not available in your city, at least reduce the amount of imported produce purchased. Buy as much local produce as possible.

When looking at food preparation, the following guidelines can be helpful.

▶ Few, if any, nutrients are lost in raw, organic foods.
▶ Drying food accounts for a loss of 9 to 14 percent of nutrients.
▶ Freezing food accounts for a loss of 10 to 24 percent of nutrients.
▶ Canning food accounts for a loss of 35 to 50 percent of nutrients.

To improve your health, move up this chain. Begin to replace canned foods with frozen foods. Replace frozen foods with dried or fresh foods. This is a process, so do what you can.

Nine—Drink Fresh Juices as Much as Possible
Juicers hit the market several years ago. Many people have a juicer tucked away in their kitchen or basement. Now is the time to pull it out. If you don't have a juicer, there are many available options. Juicers sell for as little as $30, all the way to over $300. An inexpensive *used* juicer is far better than an *unused*, expensive juicer.

Most health-food stores have juice bars. This is an excellent way to taste juices and find juices that you enjoy. It is also an excellent way to experiment when time or the appropriate machinery is not available.

There are many excellent books available on juicing. Appendix G lists some (see page 226). Unless you are eating a high percentage (50 percent or higher) of raw foods, you probably need more raw foods. Juicing is an easy way to increase our raw food consumption. Juicing also provides some excellent dietary supplements. Fresh juices become "vitamin and mineral cocktails."

"What about all of the lost fiber?" many people ask. Fiber is very important to the body. Many people asking this question are also consuming diets high in snack foods, meats, and highly processed foods. Those foods also have no fiber. To get fiber, you need to eat fruits, veggies, whole grains, and legumes. Complement your juicing with these high-fiber foods.

Processed juices do not compare to freshly made juice. Heat, chemical processing, and additives leave bottled, frozen, and canned juices with virtually no nutrients. Get out your juicer and start enjoying fresh juices.

Ten—Reduce Your Intake of Sugar!
Sugar was a big contributor to my emotional and mental problems. Most Americans consume far more sugar than they realize. When you begin to read labels, you will find that sugar, or one of its aliases, is in much of our processed foods.

What are some of the aliases of this common food? Many aliases exist for sugar, such as sucrose, dextrose, fructose, corn syrup, brown sugar, and high fructose corn syrup. Other questionable items include white grape juice, which has everything stripped out except the fruit sugar. Honey on an ingredient list is always refined honey, which is a simple sugar. If the honey is raw (which does have more nutritional benefit than refined), it will say "raw" honey on the label. Refined is always the default for a label.

White enriched flour works in the body in a similar way to sugar. Many people believe they are eating healthily by eating pasta. White-flour pasta quickly converts to sugar. It is also lacking fiber. If you choose to eat pasta, which is fine, choose pasta made from whole grains. DeBoles pasta is made from semolina and Jerusalem artichoke flour. It is a good transitional pasta for people coming off white-flour pasta. Purity Foods makes a brand of pasta by the label of VitaSpelt that is made from spelt. Spelt is a grain, with gluten, that some people with wheat sensitivities can tolerate. This pasta is much tastier than plain whole-wheat pasta, which can be fairly heavy.

I believe that white flour and white sugar are as lethal as cocaine. As much as you can, eliminate these white powders!

Americans consume over 15 times the amount of sugar that they did 100 years ago. Excessive sugar intake has been linked to arthritis, hypertension, diabetes, dental decay and, equally important, depression and fatigue.

In our efforts to cut down on sugars, we have turned to non-caloric sweeteners. The consequences of these non-caloric sweeteners have been disastrous. Nutrasweet™, for instance, is about 200 times sweeter tasting than a comparable amount of white sugar. So, by introducing saccharin and Nutrasweet™ into your body, you decrease the amount of energy in the spleen-pancreas, and the immune system is depressed.[4]

Sugar was a big contributor to my emotional and mental problems. After cleansing my body, the introduction of sugar caused immediate emotional and mental symptoms for me. Our desire for sweet is matched only by our desire for fat and salt. Reducing our sugar intake can have as many signs of withdrawal as quitting drugs.

As Dr. John Yudkin says,

If only a fraction of what is already known about the effects of sugar were to be revealed in relation to any other material used as a food additive, *that material (sugar) would be banned.*[5]

When a birthday party or celebration comes along, it is nice to have a tasty alternative to white sugar and flour. There are many sugar substitutes, not chemically based, that can be used. Use good judgment with these substitutes. The goal is still to satisfy our sweet tooth with fresh fruits.

Most Americans have turned every day into a fcast day by eating highly concentrated fat, sugar, and salt diets. Sweet treats should be just that—treats. Treats are not treats when eaten every day.

Although no sweetener at all is best for the body, if you choose to have a sweet, baked food item, it is important to know which sweeteners are less harmful. The following alternatives can produce an acceptable tasting product. The key to purchasing any product is: The less it is refined or processed, the healthier it is. Each of these products can be found in a form that is less refined than white sugar and its aliases. Here are some available sugar substitutes:

Honey. Honey is a simple carbohydrate, which means it enters the bloodstream quickly. In its processed, filtered form it should be used sparingly. Honcy is most nutritious when purchased raw and unfiltered. Refined honey will be similar to sugar, except that, being sweeter, it takes less quantity to produce a sweet dessert. Raw honey, by far the preferred, contains bee pollen (one of the most nutritious foods on earth) and bee propolis (a natural disinfectant). Buying it locally is also better. Because it is so much sweeter than sugar, you can use a much smaller quantity.

Maple syrup. Maple syrup comes from the sap of maple trees. It is also a simple carbohydrate. Purchase maple syrup that is pure and produced without formaldehyde. The packaging should say if this chemical was used. Avoid maple-flavored syrups that are mostly colored sugar water. Store pure maple syrup in the refrigerator.

Brown-rice syrup. Brown-rice syrup is a balanced sweetener, or complex carbohydrate. Balanced sweeteners enter the bloodstream slowly, reducing the sugar jacking or sugar blues associated with sugar. It is mild tasting and comes in different levels of sweetness. Because of its mild flavor, it blends well with stronger flavored sweeteners.

Sorghum or blackstrap molasses. Molasses is made from sorghum. Sorghum is a livestock-feeding plant similar to millet. Molasses is rich in potassium, iron, calcium, and the B vitamins.

FruitSource. FruitSource is a brand of sweetener. A complex sweetener, it is made from grape juice and whole brown rice. It has no artificial flavors, colors, or preservatives added. It comes in both granular and liquid forms. It can be used in baking and cooking.

Fruit Sweet. Fruit Sweet is a sweetener made by Wax Orchards. It is made from peach, pear, and unsweetened pineapple juices. Store the liquid in the refrigerator.

Sucanat. Sucanat is a brand of sweetener made from evaporated cane juice. All of the vitamins, minerals, and other nutrients found in the cane juice are retained. Only the water is removed. As a whole food sweetener, it has gone through less processing than sugar.

Stevia. Stevia is called the sweet herb. Since it is twenty-five times sweeter than honey, it should be used sparingly. Purchase it in the herb section of a health-food store. The leaf form can be used to sweeten teas. The powder form can replace sugar. Add it with the dry ingredients in cooking and baking. One-half to one teaspoon can be used for each cup of sugar.

Fruit. Ripe bananas are an excellent sweetener. Bananas can be added to muffins and cakes to increase the moisture content. When using very ripe bananas, reduce the amount of the other sweeteners, or omit them completely.

Eleven—Reduce Fats and Use Good Oils

The media has done an excellent job of educating the public of the pitfalls of too much fat. Surgeon General Koop has stated: "Of greatest concern is our excessive intake of dietary fat and its relationship to risk for chronic diseases such as coronary heart disease, some types of cancers, diabetes, high blood pressure, strokes and obesity."[6]

We know fat is bad for us. But sometimes all of the information can be a little confusing and overwhelming. Learn as much as you can about the various forms of fats. Here is my simplistic approach that works for our family.

Don't eat hydrogenated fats. These fats include margarine, shortening, and processed foods containing hydrogenated fats.

These fats work like plastic in the body. They are toxic and impossible to digest.

Use oils sparingly in cooking. We don't fry or sauté veggies in large amounts of oil. See chapter 9 for possible oil substitutes in cooking and baking.

We only use expeller pressed oils instead of solvent extracted oils. What does that mean? Most vegetable oils found in supermarkets use solvents. An example of a solvent is crude oil. The solvent is then burned off, producing a highly processed toxin. Vegetable oils may be light in color, but most are poisonous to your body.

Expeller pressed oils are made by pressing the oil from the seed, nut, or bean. No chemicals or solvents are used. Expeller pressed oils can be left unrefined, or they can be refined to produce additional stability for cooking. I prefer to use unrefined, expeller pressed oils, which have wonderful flavors. For example, corn oil adds a wonderful flavor to cornbread; since it is so much more flavorful, smaller amounts can produce excellent results. Some expeller pressed oils are organic, an even better feature. Because of their extensive research in this area and their superior products, I highly recommend Spectrum oils. They are committed to quality and education.

Store open expeller pressed oils in the refrigerator to prevent rancidity. The exception is olive oil. Quality oils should be stored unopened in cabinets away from light.

Lecithin is another oil that we use. It aids in the transmission of messages from one nerve to another, the lubrication of joints, the absorption of vitamins A and D, and the use of vitamins E and K. It can also help retard liver deterioration. Lecithin can be purchased in liquid or granular form. It is easy to add to many dishes. Store lecithin in the refrigerator.

Another excellent nutritional oil is flaxseed oil. It is nature's richest source of Omega-3 fatty acids (these essential fatty acids play a key role in maintaining the structure of the cells and in producing energy). Flaxseed oil is an alternative to fish oils, which can have pollutants from the waters the fish live in. Flaxseed oil is more stable than fish oil and costs less. Since the quality of flaxseed oil is critical to its effectiveness, I highly recommend Spectrum flaxseed oil. It is certified organic and is produced by a unique method that keeps all the seed's natural components intact.

A lecithin-canola oil mixture is good for oiling pans. Combine two parts expeller pressed canola oil with one part liquid lecithin and store this mixture in an oil spreader in the refrigerator. An oil spreader is a small container with a built-in brush. (A small airtight jar could serve as a substitute.) It's very handy for lightly oiling pans. An excellent oil spreader is made by Norpro and can be found in some kitchen-supply stores. Contact the Lifestyle for Health office (see appendix F, page 224) for further information on oil spreaders. This lecithin-canola oil mixture replaces toxic spray products. It works superbly to prepare baking or cooking pans. Food releases easily from a pan prepared with this mixture.

Twelve—Eat Whole-Grain Pastas and Breads
Many people have moved to pasta as a way to eliminate fat from their diet. They select pasta made from white enriched flour. What a waste! That type of food sticks to the intestinal tract like glue while containing almost no nutrition.

Another problem with most commercial pastas and breads is the labeling. The label might say "all natural, whole wheat," but the first ingredient on the list is white enriched flour. Again, white flour is neither a whole grain nor a wholesome product.

Read the labels. Look for products that actually use whole-grain flours. Don't be misled by the color of the product. Some bakeries use caramel coloring to simulate the natural color of whole wheat.

White flour has been robbed of its color, taste, smell, and nutrition. Not even cockroaches will eat white flour-based products. Twenty-six essential nutrients, plus the bran, have been removed from wheat to produce white flour. Four of the removed nutrients are returned (in a chemical form) to produce "enriched" flour. What an enriching process!

Whole-grain pastas and breads do exist. They are a step up

from the white-flour forms. Suggested brands of whole-grain pasta are listed in appendix C (page 204).

The next step is to begin using products with freshly milled flours. Freshly milled flour has all of the natural oils and nutrients of the grain still intact. Once the grain is ground into flour by a flour mill, the flour can be placed in the refrigerator or freezer for up to one month before the natural oils go rancid. If the freshly ground flour is left at room temperature, the natural oils will go rancid within forty-eight hours. After that time the wheat germ, comprising 90 percent of the nutrients, is also rancid. Rancid basically means that the food item has spoiled and will often smell bad. Eating rancid or spoiled food has obvious consequences, the least of which is increased toxicity to the body.

The reason to freshly mill flour is for the increased nutritional benefit to you. Natural kernels of wheat, for example, contain sixteen minerals, ten essential vitamins, plus at least four other vitamin factors generally found in bran and wheat germ. White flour is refined from the endosperm consisting mostly of starch and a small amount of protein. It contains very few vitamins and minerals. The whole grain in the flour also adds natural fiber. Freshly milled flour is also very tasty—fresh and sweet. Purchase a flour mill for easy flour milling. Information on mills can be found in chapter 10 and in appendix B (page 185).

If you choose not to mill but want quality bread, you need to find a bakery that mills its own flour. In the Rocky Mountain region, Great Harvest Bread Company produces tasty, freshly milled bread. The flavor is superb and the varieties are nearly limitless. It also sells freshly milled flour for home use.

Thirteen—Eat More Whole Grains, Legumes, Seeds, and Sprouts

When Forest and I teach on nutrition, I jokingly say, "Health food is more than just chunks of tofu and bean sprouts." Well, it is more than sprouts and tofu, but both foods, especially sprouts, are very nutritious.

Whole grains are a wonderful source of the B vitamins that help promote the health of the nerves. Whole-grain rotation (eating any one specific grain only once every three to four days) reduces the development of food sensitivities or allergies.

Wheat, the most commonly eaten grain, is high in gluten. Gluten combined with yeast is a big mucus builder. Excess mucus negatively affects the respiratory system and the colon. The most commonly cited food allergies are to wheat and gluten.

Brown rice, millet, quinoa, amaranth, oats, and barley are examples of alternate grains. Brown rice is considered a staple in health-food diets. It is high in fiber and low in fat. Brown-rice flour is an excellent thickener for sauces and gravies. It also works well with barley flour to produce quality baked items. Millet (birdseed) is the only grain that is not assimilated as an acid food in the body. Because of this trait, it is highly recommended by nutritionists. It is high in protein and rich in iron, potassium, and calcium. It is also very easy to digest. Quinoa is another round grain smaller than millet. When cooked it will expand to four times its original size. It is as high in protein as amaranth, as well as being rich in calcium, phosphorus, and iron. Quinoa flour is somewhat strong-flavored, but it works well with corn as in cornbread.

Amaranth is round and about half the size of millet. It has the highest content of protein of any of the grains. It is so nutritious that it is considered one of the key grains for the future. It is best used as a cereal or in casseroles. Amaranth flour is somewhat strong and works best in conjunction with other flours. Oats are second in protein to quinoa and amaranth. They are often considered a warming grain because of their higher fat content. They are rich in calcium, phosphorus, and iron. Barley is a light, mild grain. It is used in soups, casseroles, and as a substitute for rice. Barley flour is light and makes excellent quick breads and pie crusts. Millet, quinoa, and amaranth are considered the easiest grains to digest. Easy digestibility means that the food moves quickly through the digestive system to be assimilated by the body. It also means that the food produces little, if any, mucus and therefore does not clog the intestinal tract during elimination.

My cookbook *Lifestyle for Health* has a chapter dedicated to grains, their purpose, and methods of preparation. Experiment with different grains and cooking methods. A variety of grains in your diet will increase your natural sources of nutrients.

Other excellent books on grains include: Joanne Slatzman, *Amazing Grains* (Tiburon, CA: J. J. Kramer, Inc., 1990); Marilyn Diamond, *The America Vegetarian Cookbook from the Fit for Life Kitchen* (New York: Warner Books, 1990); Lorraine D. Tyler, *The Natural Nine* (Salt Lake, UT: Magic Mill, 1984).

Seeds help feed the brain and reproductive system. Seeds, along with nuts, do contain oil. If they are fresh and properly stored, these natural oils will not turn rancid. Buy nuts and seeds in whole form (versus chopped) for longer freshness. Store in the refrigerator or freezer.

Nut butters should not contain hydrogenated fats, added sugar, or chemicals. Almond butter is a good replacement for peanut butter. It is lower in fat, easier to digest, and higher in calcium than peanut butter.

Sprouts are germinated seeds. All of the live enzymes and nutrients contained in seeds reside in sprouts. You can purchase sprouting seeds and full-grown sprouts in health-food stores and some supermarkets.

Sprouts are easy to grow at home. You will need:

▶ Widemouthed jars—pints for a single person and quarts for a family of four
▶ Nylon net, plastic screen, or sprouting lids
▶ Dish drainer for draining jars of washed sprouts

Purchase seeds and grains from health-food stores and be sure to use organic.

The procedure for sprouting is as follows: Determine the number of seeds/grain to use by referring to the following chart. Measure seeds/grains; place in a mason jar; cover with net, screen, or sprouting lid. Rinse the seeds two or three times, then submerge them in water to an inch or two above the seeds. Set the jar upright in a warm, dark place (or cover with a dark towel). Drain after the proper soaking time—eight hours. Then rinse and drain as stated in following table. Sprouted seeds and grains can be left for a couple of hours in the sunlight to bring out the chlorophyll for additional color. Enjoy a food that is truly alive and healthy!

Seeds	Rinse and Drain	Sprouting Time	Quantity/ Yield
Alfalfa	3 x/day	3-4 days	3 Tbl. = 4 c.
Barley	3 x/day	3-5 days	½ c. = 1 c.
Beans	3 x/day	3-5 days	1 c. = 4 c.
Buckwheat	3 x/day	2-3 days	1 c. = 3 c.
Clover	3 x/day	1-2 days	1½ Tbl. = 4 c.
Garbanzo	4 x/day	2-3 days	1 c. = 3 c.
Lentils	3 x/day	3-4 days	½ c. = 3 c.
Millet	3 x/day	3-4 days	1 c. = 2 c.
Mung Bean	3 x/day	3-5 days	½ c. = 2½-3 c.
Pumpkin	3 x/day	3-4 days	1 c. = 2 c.
Brown Rice	3 x/day	3-4 days	1 c. = 2½ c.
Sesame	3 x/day	3-4 days	1 c. = 1½ c.
Sunflower	2 x/day	3-4 days	½ c. = 1½ c.

Legumes also fit into this category. Dried beans, split peas, lentils, and black-eyed peas are examples of legumes. They have little, if any, fat and are high in fiber. They are a complex carbohydrate high in vitamins and minerals. Inexpensive, legumes can be purchased in large quantities and stored in airtight containers. They will keep for at least one year. Older legumes do take longer to cook.

If you have trouble digesting legumes, try a strip of kombu. Kombu is a sea vegetable sold in dried strips. It is found in health-food stores or Asian markets. A six-inch strip adds nearly one week's worth of minerals. It also aids in the digestion of beans. Sprouting beans also helps make them easier to digest. To sprout beans, simply soak them covered in water for one day, then rinse. If time permits, soak a second day with fresh water. Cook according to directions.

I add one strip of kombu to the legumes while they're cooking. Kombu can also be added to long-cooking soups. Remove the kombu before serving, if you are hesitant to eat it. The minerals have already been deposited. Kombu is the mildest of sea vegetables and has minimal taste when cooked for long periods of time at low temperatures, as in Crockpots.

Fourteen—Reduce Your Intake of Meat
Of all the food to purchase naturally, meat is the most critical. If you choose not to follow a vegetarian diet, choose your meat wisely. We all know that poultry and fish contain less saturated fat than red meat. It is my opinion that the chemicals and steroids found in commercial meat are as serious a problem, if not more serious, than the fat content.

No government regulations exist to declare meat organic. However, there are meat producers that use no chemicals or steroids. The animals and the grains are grown without exposure to chemicals. These meats are definitely preferable to the more commonly sold meats. They are more flavorful and healthful. Many health-food stores provide this natural meat.

Fifteen—Eat Less Dairy
Dairy products are not only high in fat, but they are hard to digest. They are also the leading source of mucus. The pasteurization and homogenization processes further hinder digestibility. Pasteurization was developed to clean milk from dirty dairies and dirty handling methods. We now have clean milk that is dead.

The pasteurization process destroys the phosphates enzyme found in milk. This enzyme allows us to utilize the calcium found in milk. To determine if milk has been properly pasteurized, the milk is tested for the inactivity of the phosphates enzyme. The destruction of this enzyme renders the calcium found in milk virtually inaccessible. This doesn't take into account all of the other vitamins destroyed by heat that are rendered useless by the pasteurization process.

Some states do have raw milk and raw milk products. If the

milk source and handling methods are clean, raw milk products are easier on the digestive system than their homogenized, pasteurized counterparts. Goat's milk is easier on the human system than cow's milk. Quality goat products have a less "goaty" taste and can be quite pleasing.

Many people are concerned about getting their calcium without the use of dairy products. Many nutritional experts have addressed this issue. In a simplistic approach, a handful of sesame seeds has ten times the calcium found in one glass of milk. Tahini, a sesame-seed butter, which is equally high in calcium, can be used in salad dressings, dips, and in cooking. Figs (especially dried), almonds, seaweed, and dark green leafy vegetables are also high in calcium. Aspirin, chocolate, mineral oil, and stress can reduce the amount of calcium in the body.

Many cheese substitutes exist. Tofu cheeses have come a long way in flavor, meltability, and pricing. Tofu, with a few extra ingredients, can easily mimic cottage cheese, sour cream, and yoghurt. The new, light tofus contain less fat and no cholesterol.

Many milk substitutes also exist. Rice milk, almond milk, soy milk, and cashew cream are just a few. Nut and seed milks are easy to make at home. Recipes for nut and seed milks, and other dairy substitutes, can be found in my cookbook *Lifestyle for Health.*

Sixteen—Increase Your Water Consumption
What could be easier than to drink more water? Next to oxygen, water is the most critical factor to maintain life. The need for water cannot be overemphasized. Few people drink the daily recommendation of eight glasses.

However, drinking regular tap water is less than desirable. Tap water is very polluted. Many options for tap water exist, the easiest and least expensive of which is bottled, distilled water. Since bottled water is not regulated, care must be taken when buying it. Our nutritionist recommended distilled water as the cleanest source. It does lack some minerals, but it is without other negative factors.

The best sources of pure water are the three-stage, reverse-osmosis water-purification systems. This process provides a purer water than do simple water filters. Shaklee, Nimbus, and Water Factory Systems make available excellent water-purification systems. Ordering information can be found in appendix B, page 185.

The worst time to drink water is during mealtime. Water rushes food through the digestive system. It washes away digestive juices, including saliva, thereby interrupting digestion. Consume water one hour after meals or one-half hour before meals. Work at drinking less water during each meal.

Some people who try to drink less water during meals find they are actually thirstiest during a meal. Often the reason for this is the minimal amount of water they drink during the day. Saliva, which is the first digestive enzyme, is primarily composed of water. If a person has not consumed enough water to produce a satisfactory amount of saliva, the person will immediately become thirsty upon eating. To eliminate this problem, increase water consumption throughout the day.

Water at room temperature is also less shocking to the system. As much as possible, limit the amount of ice added to the water you consume.

Seventeen—No-No Foods to Avoid

These suggestions will lead you to improved health. Remember our philosophy: *Take one step at a time!* You do not have to carry out each of these steps immediately. You can take time to bring them into your lifestyle.

The following list contains foods that are best to eliminate, or least reduce, from your diet. Like the family we described earlier, it might take you a year to eliminate one of these foods. It is better to take a year than to never do anything.

Start where you are and begin to reduce your consumption of the products. Since many have chemicals, you might notice withdrawal symptoms. That is your body's way of saying it is dumping the toxins created by the product being reduced.

► Caffeine

► Alcohol

► Foods containing preservatives, additives, and chemicals

► High-sodium products

► MSG (monosodium glutamate) and its aliases[7]

► Food coloring

► Refined sugar, all aliases and all products using it

► White flour and all products using it

► Margarine, shortening, and high-fat products (Spectrum has a spun canola oil that is spreadable like margarine, without the hydrogenated-fat composition)

► Solvent derived oils (all expeller pressed oils will state that fact on the label)

► White rice

► Carbonated beverages

► Salt-cured or smoked foods (foods containing nitrates and nitrites)

You now have many places to begin making smarter food choices. Are you to go and do each of these suggestions tomorrow? Unless you are under the supervision and direction of a health-care practitioner—*no!* Take your time and slowly change your habits.

Each suggestion had many ways of implementation. The key is to start changing, then stay with the process. Eventually you will amaze yourself at your progress.

The next set of suggestions will help you improve your kitchen and pantry. These suggestions will support your food changes. You might even choose to implement them first. The choice is yours. Since you are a winner, you will make the choice and not be overwhelmed. You are becoming food-smart and body-healthy.

CHAPTER
EIGHT

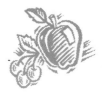

Go for the Gold

As you read our first seventeen suggestions, you may have
wondered what you should do with the rest of your environment. You don't have to take out a huge loan to change your
environment. It is possible to change in a reasonable time frame
and on a budget.

When Forest and I began our changes, we were living on
$850 a month. We used between $150 and $175 a month for
groceries. If we could make our changes on that budget, it is
possible for the average American to make changes.

We have another eight suggestions for change that will support and enhance your smarter food choices. You're on a roll;
you may as well go for the gold!

ONE—PURCHASE QUALITY COOKBOOKS

Being a cookbook author, I am aware of the importance of cookbooks. One reason I wrote three cookbooks was because I found
most health-food books unacceptable. The food was tasteless,
too difficult to prepare, and too strange to eat. The recipe names
alone intimidated and scared me.

Our family has always enjoyed having friends over to eat. When we changed our eating habits, we wondered how that would affect our social life. I found that I had a gift of converting fresh, wholesome food into tasty dishes. Even our junk-food junkie friends enjoyed eating at our home.

As many of our friends tasted health food and saw the results of our diet changes, they switched. If health food could taste this good, be affordable, and produce significant health changes, why not make the change?

Health cookbooks can make a transition much easier, less expensive, and more enjoyable for everybody. I have listed several good cookbooks in appendix H, page 229. Learn from other people's experience. Health food has come a long way from what it was in the 1960s and 1970s!

TWO—SELECT FROM A LIST OF ONE-LINERS

During my years of eating healthily, I have developed a list of one-liners. These tips and savers cover many areas. They are easy changes, once you know about them.

> ▶ *Eat slowly!* The first stage of digestion occurs in the mouth. When food is swallowed whole or only partially chewed, it puts tremendous strain on the digestive tract. Slow down and chew your food well.
> ▶ Eliminate distilled vinegar. It is good for cleaning windows, but it is toxic to your body. Raw, unfiltered vinegar aids in maintaining the pH balance of the body.
> ▶ Replace regular salt with sea salt. Sea salt has more nutritional value and much more taste. When I am without my sea salt in a restaurant, I have to use regular salt. The lack of taste is amazing. Putting regular salt on a baked potato seems to have no effect on the flavor. Sea salt is flavorful and requires only a small amount to make a significant taste change.
> ▶ Replace aluminum-based baking powder with aluminum-free powder. Rumford is a brand that has no aluminum. Aluminum is toxic to the body.

▶ Miso is a great replacement for unhealthy bouillon cubes. Miso is a fermented paste made from soybeans or other grains or nuts. Store it in the freezer or refrigerator. One tablespoon is equivalent to one bouillon cube. The lighter the color of the miso, the milder the flavor.

▶ Tahini, sesame-seed butter, is very high in calcium. It can be added to dips, soups, and baked dishes to increase calcium content. It can also add a creamy texture to soups. Start with a small quantity. Different brands vary significantly in taste. Be sure to check appendix C on preferred brands for tahini suggestions (page 204).

▶ A leaf of lettuce dropped into a pot of soup will absorb any extra oil.

▶ Store cleaned vegetable peelings and leftover veggies. These trimmings and leftovers can be used to make vegetable broth. Add water to the trimmings and simmer until the broth is flavorful. Vegetable broth can replace chicken or beef broth. Store it in the freezer in containers or in ice-cube trays.

▶ If you use expeller pressed oil to sauté veggies, heat the pan first. A hot pan will require less oil. This is especially true for woks and stir-fried dishes.

▶ Frozen fruit makes great fruit pops for kids and adults. Grapes and berries are excellent when made this way. Bananas can be frozen with or without the peels. Run frozen bananas under hot water to easily remove their peels. Frozen bananas are a great addition to fruit drinks. Blender-quick, homemade ice creams use frozen bananas. *Lifestyle for Health* and *Kid's Favorites* (two of our cookbooks) contain many recipes for fruit smoothie drinks.

▶ Instead of frying tortillas, place them in your toaster. This will toast the tortilla easily and quickly.

▶ Brown rice can be fluffy when cooked correctly. To make fluffy rice, sauté brown rice in a small amount of oil (place oil in a heated pan). When the rice smells fragrant, add the liquid. Bring mixture to a boil, lower heat to simmer, cover, and cook for about one hour. Set aside for a few minutes. This method works perfectly every time. Use twice the liquid per amount of rice. With larger quantities of rice, reduce the amount of water (for example, one cup rice to two cups water, three cups rice to five and a half cups water, etc.).

▶ Add seeds, such as sunflower and sesame, to everything. I add them to salads, muffins, and our blended morning fruit drinks. Sesame seeds contain ten times the calcium of an equivalent amount of milk. So, one-tenth of a cup (approximately four teaspoons) of sesame seeds is equivalent to one cup of milk.

THREE—DEVELOP SIMPLE, HEALTHY MENUS

A real challenge for the primary family cook is meal planning. I have dedicated chapter 10 to meal-planning strategies because of the importance of that activity.

During the transition, start changing one meal at a time. Maybe breakfasts and mornings are stressful at your house. If they are, that might not be the best meal to begin changing. Start with weekend meals. Try adding more salads to your meals.

Take some fun cooking classes to get new ideas. Get a subscription to a quality health-food magazine or newsletter for new recipe ideas. Recommended magazines and newsletters are listed in appendix F, page 224.

Getting out of the rut of food boredom is important. Finding creative, easy ways to introduce health food is crucial to your success.

FOUR—IMPROVE THE QUALITY OF YOUR COOKWARE

Dr. H. Tomlinson has done a thorough study of the effect of aluminum cookware on the body. He has published an excellent book, *Aluminum Utensils and Disease*. In his book, Tomlinson says,

I have been a medical man for forty years and because of the work I have done in relation to the aluminum question I can state, without a shadow of a doubt, and with all the urgency of my command, that the use of *aluminum in the preparation of food and food products is one the most harmful factors in modern civilization.*[1]

Aluminum cookware dissolves into our food. Research has shown that aluminum poisoning can cause many health problems; it has been linked to migraines, cancer, intestinal disorders, and Alzheimer's disease.

Many fine substitutes for aluminum cookware exist. You can use stainless steel, enamel, glass, cast-iron, and lead-free earthenware. Most commercial kitchens use aluminum, so it becomes doubly important to use the best cookware at home.

Just as aluminum cookware is toxic, so aluminum foil and aluminum foil pans are toxic. Aluminum foil has a significant reaction on tomato-based foods. When storing foods, use plastic (for example, Tupperware or Rubbermaid), glass, etc., with plastic wrap or wax paper.

FIVE—KEEP YOUR ENVIRONMENT AS CLEAN AS POSSIBLE

I had always thought that I hated cleaning because cleaning is "dirty" work. Yes, I do dislike cleaning. However, I have also learned why exhaustion hit after a day of cleaning. Most cleaning supplies are highly toxic. I have completely switched my cleaning supplies to nontoxic biodegradable cleaners. My personal preference is Shaklee. Amway is another good brand. Several alternate brands are also available in health-food stores. You will find that these alternate cleaners do not produce the toxic reactions commercial cleaners do. These cleaners are concentrated and therefore less expensive and better for our environment.

I have also switched my laundry products. Dryer sheets are a common source of skin problems. Detergents containing perfumes and heavy chemicals can also add to skin irritations. I have replaced all of those products with more gentle products. Again, I prefer Shaklee, but many other safe laundry products are on the market.

Evaluate body-care products. Avoid heavily perfumed products. Replace highly processed chemical-based products with natural ingredients. For example, most deodorants are made with alum (an aluminum derivative). As the body gets cleaner, heavy deodorants become less important. Find deodorants without alum. I prefer a deodorant by Pure & Basic called Green Tea Deodorant. Made from green tea, it is a natural deodorant. It comes in deodorant and soap forms.

Another example is common toothpaste. Most commercial toothpastes are highly fluoridated and contain sugar. Shaklee and Tom's of Maine make excellent toothpaste replacements. Our family has experienced less decay with the use of these products (along with our improved diets).

SIX—USE GOOD SENSE WHEN EATING OUT

Dining out is a challenge to any healthy lifestyle. I now take our own oil and sea salt with us. This becomes very helpful at salad and baked-potato bars. We have four or five superb health-food restaurants in Denver. We want them to stay in business, so we tell everybody about them.

Travel makes dining out a little more difficult. Check the yellow pages for health-food stores, health-food restaurants, and vegetarian restaurants. This is a starting place. Healthy snack foods go everywhere with us. We minimize temptation by taking some food with us.

For example, we take some healthier cookies (few cookies are really healthy), trail mix, or fresh fruit on our trips. When we want a snack, we have an alternative to the fast-food junk found at the gas station or airport.

We have also developed another alternative to dining out. Many of our friends now eat the way we eat. We have learned to make hospitality fun. Entertaining is too much work. So we don't do it. Instead, we have friends over and simply share a meal. What is the difference?

Entertaining means having the house clean, the table perfectly set, and at least three courses of gourmet food expertly prepared and served. My head hurts to think about such work! Hospitality is so much simpler. It means the house stays the way it is. We set the table the way we always set the table. Adding a little water to the soup, we simply share ourselves, our home, and our food with our friends. We relax and enjoy the evening.

This kind of eating is so much more enjoyable than dining out at a restaurant. I can't begin to describe how much fun we have had around our dining room table. As friends begin to reciprocate, the fun multiplies. Find some friends and learn about the lost art of hospitality.

Multiply this idea and begin to free up your cooking time. For example, find four other families to join with you. Each family could cook for one day of every week or for one week of every month for the other three families. *Voila!* You now have three free days a week or three free weeks a month. What a way to go.

SEVEN—HERBS AND SUPPLEMENTS TO THE RESCUE

Did you know that herbs are the basis of our pharmaceutical industry? Pharmaceutical companies now chemically concoct what we used to use herbs alone to do. We appreciate the significant impact herbs can make on common health problems.

We have replaced our "medicine cabinet" with an herb cabinet. Although this is a controversial subject in many places, we have found herbs to be very helpful. Our family has found the following tips to work for us. They are not prescriptions for you, merely ideas and suggestions.

Make a tea by steeping the herbs in water for five to twenty minutes. Strain the tea. If the tea is for drinking, consume it hot. If for medicinal purposes, cool before using.

► Peppermint teas, as a beverage, help to digest meals; use instead of antacids.

► Use echonecia and goldenseal for cold or flu symp-
toms. They operate as natural antibiotics.
► White willow bark and arnica have replaced aspirin as
a natural pain reliever.
► Nettles are now used as a natural antihistamine.
► Chamomile tea is a gentle sleep enhancer.
► Use aloe to relieve the pain and side effects of burns
and insect bites.

We use the following tea for eyewashes to heal pinkeye and
other eye infections.

1 teaspoon eyebright
1 teaspoon fennel seed
1 teaspoon goldenseal

Pour two cups boiling water over these herbs and let steep
until cool. Strain and use to wash the eye as needed. Store extra
in the refrigerator. Make a new mixture every one to two days.
These herbs can be purchased in bulk at health-food stores.

An herbal mixture is used for cough syrups. For deep, congested coughs:

1 teaspoon lobelia
1 teaspoon skullcap
1 teaspoon coltsfoot
1 teaspoon black cohosh
1 teaspoon licorice (powder)

Pour two cups boiling water over these herbs and let steep
until cool. Strain and drink one tablespoon every two hours, as
needed. Store extra in refrigerator. Replenish after two days.
These herbs can be found in health-food stores.

For a regular cough syrup:

1 teaspoon lungwort
1 teaspoon mullein
1 teaspoon prickly ash bark
2 teaspoons wild cherry bark

Pour two cups boiling water over these herbs and let steep until cool. Strain and drink one tablespoon every two hours, as needed. Store extra in refrigerator. Replenish after two days. These herbs can be found in health-food stores.

Many other herbal remedies exist. Brigitte Mars, a leading national herbalist and tea formulator, writes for our *Lifestyle for Health Newsletter*. She offers many courses on the benefits of herbs and can be contacted at UniTea Herbs in Boulder, Colorado. See appendix B, page 185.

Besides herbs, supplements can be helpful to the body. Remember, these are food *supplements*, not food substitutes. Food supplements are not designed to replace healthy, balanced food choices.

Many good supplements are on the market, as are many poor ones. It becomes your responsibility to determine their quality. Several factors should be considered when selecting supplements.

▶ Find out about the reputation and history of the manufacturer. What is their philosophy and goal in providing supplements?

▶ Determine how the supplements are made. Are they made from food sources or chemical sources? If chemical, you have not improved your position from using over-the-counter pharmaceuticals.

▶ Are the doses reasonable? If the label says one tablet contains megadoses of a nutrient, you can be sure that the company did not use food sources for the supplement. It is usually considered better to take more tablets of a quality source than one tablet of a poor source.

▶ Does the supplement work with other supplements? If, after a month or so, you find no change in your body, this supplement might not be right for you. I recommend that you work with a health-care provider when combining herbs and supplements. Many of them are strong and should be used with wisdom.

Herbs and supplements have been very helpful in building our bodies. We have worked at increasing our base of knowledge in this area. We now have several books on herb treatments. They provide a wide base of information on how to treat problems with herbs.

It is good to know that there are alternatives to medicine for many problems. Medicine has its place. However, it is a relief to know that many health symptoms can be effectively treated with herbs and supplements.

EIGHT—BECOME KNOWLEDGEABLE

Knowledge is an effective replacement for ignorance. When you are a victim, you are at the mercy of what the "experts" say is true. The more knowledgeable you become on health, the more responsible you can become. No expert can know your body better than you. Learn to read your body and understand its needs. When you add accurate information to those needs, you begin to develop a plan that will work for you.

We subscribe to good magazines and newsletters. We read books on health and nutrition. When classes and seminars are available, we attend. So much good material exists to help educate you on health and nutrition. Take advantage of other people's experiences. Learn from their mistakes. There is no reason to make the same mistakes that I made.

Educate yourself. Practical teaching that provides quality information to help make wise decisions is invaluable. Find teachers who have good fruit in their lives. Are the teachers healthy? If they are, then listen to what they say. Eventually you will see a pattern, and you will know that you have come across another nugget of truth.

NINE—(A FREEBIE) HAVE FUN!

Don't forget to enjoy the process. Health is not a destination, it is a lifestyle. Laugh at your mistakes. Pick yourself up, learn from your mistake, and go on. When you start to take yourself and your food choices too seriously, slow down. Team up with someone who can help you laugh. A merry heart does as much good as medicine.

Enjoy yourself. Food is not spelled s-e-r-i-o-u-s. It is spelled l-i-f-e. Learn to eat that you may live an abundant life. We don't live to eat. We eat that we may live with health and not dis-ease.

CHAPTER
NINE

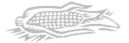

Reform Your Kitchen and Pantry

W e all know the saying "Time is money."
Consider the truth of that statement as you start changing your pantry and kitchen. If you want to save time you may need to spend some money. If you want to save money you will need to spend some time. However, there are many ways to manage that money and time expenditure so that it is reasonable and affordable.

The speed with which you convert your pantry and kitchen is influenced not only by your money but also by your ability to adapt to new tools. Kitchen gadgets are a waste of money and space if they sit unused in a cabinet. Pantry conversions are worthless if you never use the new contents of the pantry.

It is important that you customize these ideas into a plan that will work for you and your family. As I had the money and as I ran out of unhealthy food, I replaced it with a new, healthy choice. Slowly but surely, I replenished my pantry and home with healthy products. Over time I added kitchen appliances that made cooking fun and easy. The results are tasty meals that please all of us and keep me on schedule and within my budget.

As you decide to use different products in your home, take

the time to find out what you are currently using. To do this, take an inventory of your pantry, cleaning basket, laundry room, and medicine cabinet. That will take time, so allow yourself that time. Pick the area you most want to change. Inventory one area at a time.

Most people think the first area to address should be the pantry. However, changing cleaning and laundry products may be a much simpler step. Using a toxic-free cleaner in place of a toxic cleaner is a simple change. That might be the place for you to start.

PANTRY CONVERSIONS

The following items are found in my pantry. As you run out of your current food items, check this list as a guideline. Items on the left are found in the standard pantry; items on the right are found in a healthier pantry. Switch your stock over as you can afford to, both financially and mentally.

You may not be familiar with some food items. A brief description for unusual foods can be found in the glossary. Brand suggestions can be found in appendix C (page 204).

Pantry Items

baking powder	aluminum-free baking powder
biscuit mixes	whole-grain mixes
black tea	herbal tea
bouillon cubes	miso (store in refrigerator) pure vegetable bouillon
cereals	use whole-grain hot or cold cereals; avoid cereals with additives, sugar, hydrogenated fats, or white flour
chips	look for organic, low-salt, and baked chips corn or tortilla chips blue-corn chips

	bean chips
	brown-rice chips
	vegetable chips
coffee	herbal teas
distilled vinegar	apple-cider vinegar
	brown-rice vinegar
	umeboshi-plum vinegar
nuts and seeds	preferably raw, store in refrigerator or freezer
	almond butter (instead of peanut butter)
	almonds
	cashews and cashew butter
	canola seeds
	pecans
	sesame seeds
	sunflower seeds
	walnuts
pancake mixes	whole-grain mixes
pork and beans	the following beans can be purchased dried or canned:
	adzuki beans
	black beans
	black-eyed peas
	garbanzo beans
	kidney beans
	lentils
	lima beans
	navy beans
	pinto beans
	refried beans
	split peas
salt	sea salt
	Real Salt (brand name)

	salt-free seasonings such as Parsley Patch
saltine crackers	whole-grain crackers rice cakes honey grahams (with whole-grain flours and no sugar)
shortening	expeller pressed oils (keep in refrigerator) canola oil corn oil olive oil sesame oil walnut oil
spices and herbs	allspice basil bay leaves cardamon cayenne celery salt chervil chili powder cinnamon cloves cumin curry dill weed fennel seeds garlic powder ginger marjoram mustard (dry) nutmeg onion powder oregano paprika

	parsley
	poultry seasoning
	red pepper flakes
	rosemary
	sage
	summer savory
	tarragon
	thyme
	turmeric
soups	look for enamel-lined cans and soup mixes without chemicals
soy sauce	tamari
vegetable oil	expeller pressed oils (keep in refrigerator)
	canola oil
	corn oil
	olive oil
	sesame oil
	walnut oil
white bread	whole-grain bagels
	whole-grain bread
	whole-grain muffins
	whole-grain pita bread
	whole-grain tortillas
	unleavened, sprouted bread
white flour	whole-wheat flour
	whole-wheat pastry flour
	barley flour
	buckwheat flour
	cornmeal (yellow, white, blue)
	kamut flour
	spelt flour
white pasta	artichoke pasta
	vegetable pastas

	udon or soba pasta (Asian pastas) whole-grain pasta (homemade or purchased)
white rice	brown rice wild rice whole-rice blends amaranth barley couscous kasha millet quinoa packaged whole-grain mixes (pilafs, tabouli, etc.)
white sugar	raw, unfiltered honey maple syrup (store in the refrigerator) brown-rice syrup FruitSource molasses Sucanat

Refrigerator Items

cheese	raw milk cheese tofu cheese almond cheese

eggs	farm-fresh, fertile eggs
	    (found in health-food stores)
	tofu
	egg replacer
	yo cheese
	Fantastic Foods (brand name)
	    tofu scrambler

juices	freshly made juices sugar-free, real fruit juices, no additives

margarine	expeller pressed oils (keep in refrigerator) canola oil corn oil olive oil sesame oil walnut oil
meat	organic meats tofuburger mixes or frozen burgers seiten meat alternatives tempeh meat alternatives tofu
milk	bovine-free raw milk (from a clean source) raw goat's milk (from a clean source) almond milk cashew cream rice milk soy milk
sauces and condiments	sugar-free ketchup eggless mayonnaise preservative-free salad dressings preservative- and sugar-free mustards salsa fruit-only jams
vegetables	organic, if possible (see vegetable list in chapter 7)

BULK BUYING

A way to save money when buying health food is bulk buying. Usually this is done through wholesale buying or buying in large quantities. When you buy wholesale, you can realize 20 to 40 percent savings on your food costs. Many food items easily lend

themselves to buying in bulk. However, you must consider a
few key items before embarking upon such a plan.

1. Bulk buying requires up-front cash. If your cash flow is
   tight, you may need to plan to make such an expenditure
   over a few months. Once you get into the cycle of
   buying in bulk on a bimonthly or monthly basis, you
   will probably wonder why you ever shopped weekly.
2. Bulk buying requires storage containers and storage
   space. If you have a very small living space, you must
   become very creative in your storage-space selection or
   you may not want to bulk-buy.
3. Be sure you like the item you bulk-buy. It doesn't matter
   how great a buy an item is; if your family doesn't
   like it, it was a poor decision. Be sure to try a product
   before bulk-buying (unless you like to give food away).
4. Buy what you use and use what you buy. Be sure you
   bulk-buy foods that you need and use. If you don't
   need a case of rice milk, don't bulk-buy it.

Food-buying clubs can be a great way to save money, if they
are well-run. I was in a club that operated out of a spirit of poverty
and disorganization. Each month the club was "short" about one
hundred dollars. By the time we paid our portion of the shortage,
we overpaid for our food.

I have been in my current food-buying club for over three
years and find it an easy way to save money. If you are not in
one, you may want to consider starting one. If possible, I highly
recommend that you become part of a well-run club before starting
your own. Companies that are open to wholesale buying and
food-buying clubs can be found in appendix B, page 185.

FOOD STORAGE

I have bought many containers, from Tupperware and
Rubbermaid to less expensive brands. Canning jars, bags, and
even plastic buckets from grocery-store bakeries will work.

My budget and my desire for order dictate the option I select. The most important factors to me are visibility (how easy it is to see the contents) and usability (how easy it is to pour, scoop, etc.). Look at any container as a possible resource for food storage. Jars are a great way to store tea bags. Baskets can store medicinal herbs. Garage sales are a great source of large containers.

HELPFUL APPLIANCES

Having the right tool makes any job easy. Having the right tool for cooking makes cooking much more enjoyable. The more I cook, the more I enjoy my kitchen gadgets. They save me time, and more important, they keep me cooking. As you can imagine, my family likes to see me cook.

I have found several different appliances to be of help in the kitchen. I have added them over time as I have had the money, desire, and interest. None of them is a necessity except maybe my blender. However, as much as I cook, I enjoy each of them. Buying information for this equipment can be found in appendix B, page 185.

Wok

When purchasing a wok, I highly recommend a good quality stainless steel wok that can be placed directly over a burner (electric or gas). I find that clectric woks do not get hot enough. Also, the Teflon interior flakes and is not a healthful finish for any pan.

Blender

Blenders are invaluable in making fruit smoothies (our breakfast staple). They are also helpful in making homemade dressings and many other foods. If possible, get a blender with a high-grade motor or as an attachment to a good food center (for example, Bosch, Oster, or Kitchen Aid).

Seed Grinder

Seed grinders are great to grind seeds and nuts into fine pieces, powders, or butters. We use ours to grind seeds and nuts for cooking and baking. A high-powered blender, such as a Bosch, can grind seeds and nuts. If you do not have a seed grinder, a clean coffee grinder will also do the job.

Steamer

You can get inexpensive metal basket steamers to set in pans for steaming. You can also get the large electric steamers. I personally prefer my big electric steamer. It is easy to clean, it automatically shuts off (no more burned pans from the water evaporating), and it holds an adequate amount of produce. The electric steamers can also be used to steam grains.

If you have neither, you can place bamboo steamers on top of boiling water in a wok. This method allows for steaming many different dishes, one in each bamboo basket.

Salad Spinner

A salad spinner is a great manual device used to spin-dry greens (lettuce, fresh herbs, etc.). This helps you to quickly dry greens. Dried greens will deteriorate slowly, thereby lasting longer. They also make a crisper salad.

Tortilla Maker

This is a luxury. Since we don't eat much wheat, having the option of spelt or barley tortillas is wonderful. Homemade tortillas are far superior to commercially prepared tortillas. The variety and quality options make this a fun device.

Pasta Machine

This has become one of my favorite machines. Homemade, fresh pasta is far superior to packaged. It also allows you to control the ingredients—the quality and the type of flour used. Once you switch, you will never go back.

Bread Machine

A bread machine gives you the luxury of having homemade bread easily and quickly. Simply toss the ingredients into the container. The machine does the rest of the work, from mixing to kneading to baking. It makes one loaf of bread at a time. Be sure to look for a machine that effectively handles whole-grain flour. As with any electric machine, the power of the motor is key.

Kitchen Center

A kitchen center is a combination of many appliances in one. It contains a powerful base with mixers, blenders, food processors, and other available attachments. It is versatile, cost-effective, and easy to use. My favorite kitchen center is a Bosch, a very powerful machine that allows you to make and knead twelve to twenty-four pounds of dough at once. It also provides a base for a blender, a slicer, a juicer, and many other attachments. If you are looking for a complete food center, I highly recommend a Bosch. This machine will last you a lifetime.

Pizza Stone and Paddle

If you eat pizza on a regular basis, this is really a great buy. It will help you make crispy pizza easily and quickly. Whether the pizza is homemade (the best!) or frozen, a pizza stone will produce a superior product. It will also turn your oven into a hearth oven that produces excellent cookies and breads.

Crockpot

What a time saver for busy days! I use my Crockpot often during the winter for soups or to prepare stock from leftover vegetable trimmings or chicken wings and backs. It is regularly used to cook beans and some grains. I personally prefer the ones with removable containers for ease of cleanup. This type provides a more even heat distribution to the food. I do not recommend the ones with Teflon finish.

Juicer

Juicers have also become a staple appliance in our daily food-preparation process. We have both an expensive one (Omega) and an inexpensive one. The inexpensive one does a quick glass of carrot juice during the day. Our heavy-duty juicer is better for leaf vegetables, pineapples, and quantity juicing.

If you are looking for a juicer but are not sure you will use it, you might want to consider a less expensive one. If you find that you really enjoy juicing, you can always purchase a more expensive one later. We enjoy having both juicers.

Dehydrator
Dehydrators are great for drying extra produce from the summer. Vegetables can be dried for soups and for soup mixes. Dried fruit makes excellent snacks, if eaten in moderation. Dehydrators make inexpensive fruit leather and jerky (beef, turkey, or even salmon). They also dry herbs and flowers.

Canner
I have a canner but rarely use it to can anything but my homemade salsa. Canned produce loses its nutrients, so I do not recommend canning as a way to preserve the bulk of your produce. Eating seasonally allows you to keep food costs down, while still having fresh produce. Fresh is always better than canned. Freezing and drying are preferred to canning.

Flour Mill
This is a wonder appliance to grind your own flour. Freshly ground flour has all of the natural oils intact. Flour with rancid oils tastes bitter and may account for some reactions to baked foods. Whole grains are inexpensive. It takes about five minutes to grind fifteen cups of grain. Store freshly milled flour for up to one month in the refrigerator or freezer.

Salad Shooter
I use a salad shooter more frequently than my large food processor. It is easier to use, store, and clean. It's a big help for quick grating jobs, such as salads, nuts, etc.

Pressure Cookers
Pressure cookers allow you to cook beans in about twenty minutes. Many meals can be prepared in less than thirty minutes. Soups take about ten to twenty, and chicken can be "fried"

without oil in about eight. These are real time savers. Be sure to purchase pressure cookers with safety-release features.

Freezer/Refrigerator

I have found an extra refrigerator to be a big help. You can easily pick one up at a garage sale. It will accommodate all of the extra produce you will be eating and will come in especially handy during the summer and holidays.

I try to make extra food (muffins, casseroles, etc.) and freeze them. A large freezer is invaluable for this purpose and for the storage of freshly milled flours.

⸺

Remember, we have been adding these appliances over the years. I managed quite well without many of them. To be effective, they must save time and help keep cooking fun. Otherwise they are a waste of money and a "white elephant" in your house. Remember, you get to decide what you do and when you do it.

When you cook at home as much as we do, these appliances add to the fun of cooking. They also help me add variety and creativity to our meals. This is so important to prevent boring meals. It also helps prevent burnout of the cook.

CHAPTER
TEN

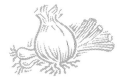

Meal Planning

How often have you heard or spoken the following words: "What's for dinner?"

I'm sure millions of houses echo with those words every night. Many American families come home from work tired. They gobble "stuff," mistakenly assumed to be food, while relaxing in front of the television. Then they rush to the next activity in their fast-paced life. Just reading those words can make a person tired.

In the past I lived a life just as hectic as that description, if not more so. The presence of food merely quieted my roaring stomach. Meals were a constant hassle. For years I tried to hire a "wife" to take care of my home and cook my meals. I fully understand a fast-paced life filled with schedules overflowing from money and time demands. Convenient anything seemed a necessity for survival.

NOURISHING MEALS

Is there an alternative? Yes. Does it require being home twenty-four hours a day? No. Slowly but surely, we have developed nourishing meals. As a family, we plan our meals and enjoy the results. It has taken time and commitment, but mealtime is now our favorite time of the day. We leave the table nourished in every area of our life. Yes, there is an option.

Let me describe a typical meal at our home, whether it is just the three of us or a dinner with others.

—

Friends (or just the three of us) come into our home, to relax and enjoy some tasty food. The meal begins when they (or we) walk in the door to a peaceful, orderly environment. What a haven that represents in this harried world!

We sit down to an attractive table with place mats, napkins, and candles. Yes, we eat by candlelight nearly every meal. A mouthwatering aroma tantalizes our taste buds.

Here comes the food. It appeals to our eyes with a rainbow of colors. As the food enters our mouths, we experience the texture, taste, and nourishment of real food.

Conversation hums around the food. We laugh and take our time. Mmmm, what a meal!

—

Is that our normal mealtime, or the exception? That is our normal mealtime. It may just be the three of us. Or, it may be with some friends. Some of you may say, "That's a utopia. That's impossible for a normal family like us. We have more kids and a tougher schedule." That's a reasonable response.

This word picture contains many elements that we will discuss in this chapter. One or two of the elements may not work for your family, but I'm sure that you will find a few to be helpful wherever you are. As you share these ideas with your family, enlist their help. Working toward a satisfying mealtime is something that every member can participate in.

As the old saying goes, "Don't throw out the baby with the bath water." Find the pieces that work for you, or that you would like to see operate during your mealtime. Just as with the healing process in general, you have a lifetime to make these changes.

No one will be upset with you if you implement a few of these ideas over time.

Occasionally, our schedule does not allow for such a relaxed meal. However, when I notice the fast pace beginning to regularly steal our relaxation from us, I know it is time to prune the schedule. We value this time of peace and relaxation, so we diligently guard and protect it.

Our commitment to family relaxation is a joint decision and a high priority to each of us. Because it is a family decision, we are each responsible to see that we stick to it. When we start to slip, one us holds the rest of us accountable. We're not trying to do this by ourselves. We are doing it as a family.

Meal planning is more than a quickly devised grocery list or spontaneous trip to the store. It includes all of the activities necessary to produce an environment and an experience of relaxation and nourishment. Producing that experience on a regular basis is a process that takes time and practice.

Are your mealtimes like our opening description? Or, is your fast food quickly eaten while watching television? If so, you have some wonderful opportunities ahead of you.

You may not want a format like ours. Maybe you just want to improve a little bit. That is okay. Allow yourself time to make the changes you and your family want to make. Take one step at a time. A pleasant surprise awaits you. Mealtimes can be fun.

MEAL INGREDIENTS

What are the components of a meal? As I have examined our mealtime, I have noticed that we have some components that many people totally overlook. Some components represent areas of struggle, such as menu planning.

Preparing the environment for a meal is akin to preparing the mind for health. Just as the environment surrounding our meal affects our meal, so our mind affects our food choices and decisions. Take time to develop the atmosphere surrounding your meals. A simple meal eaten in a relaxing, quiet environment is worth far more than a gourmet banquet eaten in the midst of strife and confusion.

The following components affect meals. They represent the skeleton upon which we build a whole, satisfying meal and, consequently, a healthy body. Whether you have two hours to plan a meal or just a few minutes, these ingredients can be added as you choose. It takes commitment to produce this kind of mealtime. With practice it becomes easier and easier. These components include:

► Environment
► Table setting
► Tasty, nourishing food
► Food presentation
► When to eat what
► Sounds
► Knowledge of food
► Meal planning

Each of these factors is involved in every meal we eat, whether we are aware of it or not. Mealtime represents a time to feed the whole person. Our body, the five senses, our mind, our emotions, and our spirits want nourishment during meals. When we do not feed each area, we experience some form of malnutrition.

In this chapter we will discuss the components of an ideal meal. You can decide which will work for you. We will also discuss the best times to eat and the best combinations of food. Timing and combining maximize the efficiency of the body. Knowing the barriers to effective meal planning is the first step to overcoming those barriers. Saving time and money is the desire of every meal provider, so we will address knowledge and planning. Finally, we will present specific meal-planning techniques for breakfasts, lunches, snacks, desserts, feasts, and dinners.

From grocery lists to grocery shopping, we will make running a kitchen a smoother, simpler project. There is even an overview on fasting. Fasting is an easy way to do a mini-cleanse and keep that stubborn appetite under control.

As we discuss each of these areas, your awareness of its impact on a meal will increase. The way you choose to handle each ingredient becomes a personal matter. The key is to become aware of these factors and begin to consciously include them in your meal. Manage your meal instead of being a victim to meal-time.

MEAL ENVIRONMENT

I have found that the orderliness of the environment surrounding the eating area does affect digestion. An orderly environment is not a sterile, perfectly cleaned, dead environment; it is peaceful and alive, with everything in its place. It is emotionally relaxed and physically comfortable.

A strife-filled home is a home out of order. It is a quick way to produce indigestion. Food does not digest in the midst of strife. Strife is manifested through quarrels and tension. As much as possible, make a family decision to eliminate strife. Particularly avoid strife during meals. Make meals as peaceful as possible.

During different seasons in your life, peace will look and sound different. Infants and toddlers add a whole new dimension to mealtime. Teenagers offer another aspect to scheduling meals. Take the season in stride. Be versatile with the demands of each season. Don't expect your toddler to use a napkin. Include older children in conversation. The old adage "Children are to be seen and not heard" does not promote order or a healthy meal for the child.

Revise it as your seasons change. Encourage peace and relaxation. Keep the table and surrounding areas as orderly as possible. As you begin to address each of the other meal factors, you will automatically be affecting your environment.

SET THE TABLE

As a former home economics teacher, I am aware of the "proper" way to set a table. However, in this section I am not addressing proper table setting. Certain table additions, however, can add to a relaxed environment. Just as the right accessory to a garment can "make" the look, so a table accessory can "make" the meal.

Many families never even eat at a table. They eat standing up in the kitchen or in front of a television. In that setting, food is a nuisance. It is quickly inhaled so that the next important activity can be pursued. That approach ignores the importance of digestion.

A table serves to bring a family together. It becomes a physical symbol of togetherness and nurturing. When possible, use a table for meals. It doesn't matter if you use a formal dining room table or a cozy kitchen bench. Sometimes we set a tablecloth on the floor in front of our fireplace and have a picnic. Often, we eat in our dining room. Other times we eat in the kitchen. The location or grandeur of the table is not as critical as the table itself. Select a table that is comfortable for you.

At the age of six or seven, our daughter had the job of setting the table. She learned how to coordinate place mats and napkins. The silverware and plates were placed on the table. One of her favorite table additions was and is candles. Children, big and little, enjoy eating by candlelight. Candlelight relaxes and soothes. We often eat by candlelight. Buying candles on sale for a quarter a candle makes this a small investment with a big return.

Even if you choose not to use place mats and napkins, at least take a few minutes to put the plates and silverware on the table. This helps extend a visual invitation to the meal. It says, "Dinner is ready!" What a welcoming sight! We often set the table for the next meal as we clean off the dishes from the current meal.

EAT NOURISHING, TASTY FOOD

As important as the environment is, nothing can replace the satisfaction of a delicious, nutritious meal. As enjoyable as dining out can be, the best meal is still a flavorful home-cooked meal. The rich aroma of homemade soup mingling with the hearty fragrance of homemade bread is impossible to deny.

Learning how to prepare health food that tastes good is

important. It doesn't matter how healthy food is; if the food tastes lousy, no one will eat it. Surrounding yourself with good cookbooks and cooking knowledge is essential.

If cooking is taking too much time, you probably are not planning your meals, or you are using ineffective cooking methods. Knowing which methods to use can greatly reduce the time spent in a kitchen. Later in this chapter we will address both cooking methods and techniques for preparing simple, nutritious meals. Health food should be some of the tastiest, most attractive food you have ever eaten, and cooking is an acquired skill that anybody can master.

Learn to savor each bite of food that you place in your mouth. So often we gobble our food, totally unaware of its flavor. Take the time to chew the food so that the flavors explode in the mouth. Mouthwatering flavor comes from smell, taste, and texture. Rushing that process reduces the full impact of the food to your taste buds.

FOOD PRESENTATION

As a cooking instructor, I am convinced that people eat with their eyes as much as with their mouths. In a recent cooking class, I made a simple black bean soup, placed it between a two-layered pizza crust, and topped it with salsa. When I unmolded that "pizza" on a tray and surrounded it with variegated greens and cherry tomatoes, I had a culinary masterpiece. The food was simply bread and an inexpensive bean soup. The presentation made it a masterpiece.

As a rule, I never set a pan on the table. I know I dirty extra dishes by placing the food into bowls and onto platters. The extra dirty dishes are worth the visual impact. Beautifully presented food tastes better. Taking the time to beautifully serve the food tells my family that they are important.

Adding a touch of parsley or placing cooked veggies around broiled chicken is a simple thing to do. Yet, the result is far-reaching. Simple fare becomes special, and each person feels honored.

When I serve cake (yes, we do eat cake—whole-grain and sugar-free, of course) to our friends, it is served on a tray. It is amazing how much further a cake can go when served this way. A few fresh strawberries or a fresh flower add a bright touch to a dessert tray.

Inadvertently, people smile when they see such a beautiful presentation. Beauty is in the eye of the beholder. The eye looks for beauty. It is fun to behold beautiful food, especially when it is in front of you and for you. When that food is healthy and tasty, who can resist?

TIMING IS EVERYTHING!

Knowing when to eat is as important as setting aside enough time to eat. The body operates on a schedule, whether we are aware of it or not. That clock leads the body into performing certain activities. That body cycle is shown below.

▶ 4:00 a.m. to 12:00 p.m. is elimination time. During this time body waste and food debris are eliminated. It is best to eat only fruits during this time. Fruits quickly digest and therefore minimally affect the elimination process.

▶ 12:00 p.m. to 8:00 p.m. is appropriation time. Eating and digestion occur during this time. Fruits, veggies, proteins, and starches, in proper combinations, are eaten during this time.

▶ 8:00 p.m. to 4:00 a.m. is assimilation time. Food is absorbed and used during this part of the cycle. Food should not be eaten at this point.

All of us have eaten a late-night meal. The next morning we feel extremely fatigued. The reason is because during the night time cycle (8:00 p.m. to 4:00 a.m.), the body is supposed to be absorbing nutrients and repairing the system from daily wear and tear.

Eating during this period robs the body of the energy necessary to absorb and digest nutrients. Digestion is a very energy-intensive mechanism. The body has little time for healing and rest while it's digesting. When the body has to digest food during this digestion-absorption cycle, the person will feel tired.

Since digestion requires so much energy, we need for it to occur as efficiently and effectively as possible. This is where proper food combination is helpful. If foods are poorly combined, digestion can take up to eight hours to complete. Properly combined food requires as little as three hours. This represents tremendous time and energy savings to the body. Proper food combinations provide us with more energy, mental clarity, and emotional stability, and an ability to handle stress better.

Improper food combinations result in energy loss, enzyme depletion, and toxicity. Food putrefies in the intestines, which leads to gas, bloating, and poor elimination. All these results lead to sickness, excess weight, and dis-ease.

Food combining can be as intricate or as simple as you make it. I have simplified food combining into a couple of guidelines. Remember, these are guidelines, not laws carved in stone. Work toward consistency, and ignore the temptation to become frustrated.

1. Eat fruit twenty to thirty minutes before a meal or two to three hours after a meal. Melons should be eaten by themselves.
2. Never combine a protein and starch or two different proteins. Protein can be eaten with nonstarchy vegetables. Starch can be eaten with vegetables.

Examples of protein are beans, nuts, seeds, and meat. Starches are potatoes, grain, pasta, and winter squash. An exception is beans. Although a protein, they can be combined with starches (for example, beans and rice). Beans also include all soy products (tofu, tempeh, etc.).

If you're not a vegetarian, eat meat with salads or nonstarchy vegetables. Otherwise, eat a baked potato with veggies instead of meat. Eat veggie sandwiches instead of meat-and-bread sandwiches. Use meat-free sauces on pasta.

These combinations may take some time to implement in your life. Being aware of them is the first step. I found that good food combining also helped in my weight loss and weight stability. I did not have to sacrifice certain foods. Instead, I learned when and in what combinations to eat these foods.

In addition to acknowledging our body clock and proper food combining, we must take time to eat. I remember many meals consumed in minutes because I was in a hurry. Today, I refuse to eat if I have to rush a meal too quickly. Fast-food restaurants promote fast eating. People pay the price of fast eating with indigestion and fast dis-ease. Take time to eat, chew, and thoroughly enjoy your food.

LISTEN TO THE SOUNDS

Conversation and quiet music can provide tremendous value to any meal. Have you ever noticed that a five-star restaurant rarely has a crying baby or a television playing in the background? People pay large amounts of money for "ambience." You can create that ambience by managing the noise surrounding your mealtime.

I often have soft background music playing during dinner. That music works like a metronome. It sets a quiet, slow pace for the meal. Music relaxes and soothes us.

Conversation at a meal can be an asset or a liability. Many of America's business deals are consummated around a dinner table. Dinner conversation can reflect high-powered business deals or intimate dinners for two.

Sadly, at home, many of us sit at a meal with nothing to say. Let mealtime be a time of learning conversation skills. Talk to each other. Ask questions. Learn to listen. This is a wonderful opportunity to let others know that you are interested in their day's activities and in them. Getting someone to talk at a meal can be as simple as asking a question. "Tell me about your day." Children, spouses, and guests respond to such a question.

Conversation extends the time within which a meal is eaten. This extra time allows the body to adequately chew and digest the food. Do not underestimate the value of communication. It not only builds healthier relationships, it builds healthier bodies.

MEAL PLANNING

Have you ever noticed that a professional skater can make skating look so simple? However, balancing on those ridiculously small blades is nearly impossible for the novice! To try to duplicate the professional's intricate moves is impossible. Why? The professional has years of practice added to his or her knowledge.

The next section will give you the knowledge you need to produce quality meals. You provide the practice sessions. A combination of this knowledge and your practice will produce meals that are nourishing and enjoyable for you and your family.

Practice in my life has produced a healthier body for me and my family. Eating has once again become fun, productive, and enjoyable. Take some time and enjoy the process of creating nourishing, tasty, relaxed meals.

The first step to meal planning is knowing what to eat. We have discussed twenty-five ways to make smarter food choices (in chapters 7 and 8). What is the goal of these choices? The goal is to eat the food that produces the most health possible.

Most Americans know they eat too much protein, fat, and sugar. Many nutritionists consider the average diet to be composed of:

▶ 20 percent complex carbohydrates
▶ 45 percent fat
▶ 15 percent protein
▶ 18 to 20 percent sugar

That breakdown represents excess fat, sugar, and protein. It shows a lack of simple and complex carbohydrates. Complex carbohydrates include starchy vegetables, sprouts, whole grains, beans, and legumes. Simple carbohydrates include fruits and nonstarchy vegetables. Starchy vegetables include black-eyed peas, corn, green peas, lima beans, parsnips, potatoes, rutabagas, turnips, and winter squash.

As much as possible, work toward a diet of 70 percent fruit and vegetables. The more they are eaten in a raw form, the better. The remainder of the diet can be grains, protein sources, and fat. As you eat a diet rich in carbohydrates, you will automatically increase your fiber, while reducing your sugar and fat content. Following the suggestions found in chapter 7 will cause you to increase your intake of healthier foods.

I have found it better to focus on what to eat instead of what to avoid. People's minds resist the word *don't*. When we see a sign that says "Don't touch, wet paint," we are tempted to reach out to touch it. When we say "Don't eat this or that," we immediately want that food more than any other food.

Instead of saying "I *shouldn't* eat fat, sugar, and too much protein," try saying, "I *want* to eat food that will feed my body." Do you notice a difference? Learn to eat a diet rich in vegetables and fruits. Experience the benefits of whole, natural foods. Your body will quickly respond to these foods.

Knowledge is helpful, but it does not replace effort. Healthy, nutritious meals require effort on your part. Take one piece of information at a time and add it to your daily routine. Then add another piece. Each addition will bring you closer to your goal of a healthy meal feeding a healthier body.

So often we look for health to be a complex and "deep" issue. Yet, over and over we see that health is a simple truth. Health is as simple as what we eat, how we think, and what we do. Living in health is where the effort and work begin.

At this point you know enough to become healthier. The next phase requires your participation. Life-giving knowledge will rot if hidden away on a bookshelf. Knowledge dies if it remains a vague memory in your mind. Only you can breathe life into knowledge by living it. Begin to apply what you know.

There is a critical phase between getting knowledge and applying it. That step is planning. It is the step most overlooked in the area of meals. We know the saying, "When we fail to plan, we plan to fail."

Why do we ignore planning our meals? We know we should

plan, but we don't. Somehow, five o'clock and dinnertime rolls around too quickly day after day. We complain that

▶ cooking takes too much time.
▶ we don't know how to cook.
▶ our meals are boring.
▶ planning takes too much time.

And the list goes on and on. Do any of these complaints sound like you? Complaining is the sign of victimitis. If you want to go beyond being a victim, you have to take responsibility for the meal as much as for the food choices. A winner says, "I am going to learn how to prepare nutritious, tasty meals." I can give you the techniques, but you have to decide to employ them.

Planning meals with traditional menu-planning methods can be unbearably time-intensive. That is why I worked at developing simple, quick techniques. Planned meals mean I have, on hand, the necessary ingredients to prepare several meals. I eliminate unnecessary trips to the store, frustrations from not having the right foods, and boring leftovers. Planning simplifies life.

The meal-planning techniques I will present shortly can help you know what to cook. Waiting until the last minute only shrinks the available options to the contents of your refrigerator. Learning effective planning techniques opens an entire grocery store of options for a meal.

Boring meals come from boring cooks. So, how can a boring cook become creative? Surround yourself with creative cookbooks and pictures of alluring meals and vary the food based on the season. A variety of ingredients, even prepared with similar methods, will add a spark of interest to any "old" menu.

The big, legitimate stumbling blocks to meal planning are time and money. When we are short of either, we eliminate planning. In reality, that is when we most need to plan. Let's take a look at some time and money savers.

TIME AND MONEY SAVERS

Beans and grains are some of the least expensive foods available. During the time we spent $150 a month for our family of three for groceries, I prepared many bean and grain dishes. Beans can be used in soups, on salads, and in many popular ethnic dishes. Grains can be cooked, sprouted, or baked. Both foods are filling, substantial, and inexpensive. They can be purchased in cans and can be cooked in crockpots or in other quick ways, such as quick-cooking brown rice.

Buy produce seasonally. Fruits and veggies should represent at least half of our diet. Buying them seasonally can drastically affect our food budget and variety. Produce prices can vary by 50 to 100 percent from store to store. If produce represents half of your budget, you can see how quickly the savings can mount. For example:

Food	In Season	Out of Season	Price Difference
asparagus	$.99 pound	$2.49 pound	250%
melons	$.29 pound	$.99 pound	340%

We rarely choose to spend two to three times a normal price for clothing. Yet, many people casually overpay by these huge amounts weekly for produce. Produce varies more than any other grocery-store product.

Read the weekly produce specials in your local newspaper. Weekly produce specials influence my menu planning and grocery shopping. Knowing produce seasonality and prices affects your budget.

I have overheard people say, "That fruit is too expensive to buy." Yet, at the check-out stand, their cart is piled high with snack and dessert items. Those items (high in fat and void of nutrition) totaled much more than the "expensive" fruit. We have to retrain our minds when it comes to food expenditures. Saving money on unhealthy foods frees money to be spent on healthier, smarter food choices.

Many grocery stores have a section of "slightly imperfect" produce. This is produce sold at reduced prices for quick sales. I have found many good buys with this produce. It is often exactly what I need for a soup, salad, or casserole.

Knowing the people in the produce section of your market will help you find out what is available. Once, while Forest was talking to a produce manager, he discovered they were throwing out "imperfect" bananas. The only problem with these bananas was some slits in the skin. Forest left the store with fifty pounds of *free* bananas. At home, we promptly bagged the bananas and froze them. They were perfect for fruit smoothies (our morning fruit drinks) and baking.

During the summer and fall, local farmers' markets are a great source for affordable, fresh produce. Often, local produce has fewer chemicals. (Be sure to check the source of the produce. Some vendors buy imported produce to sell at these markets.)

If the produce is local, it has been allowed to ripen and is much better tasting than commercial produce. Farmers' markets are usually listed in the newspapers during the summer and fall seasons. Prices are usually less than in the grocery stores.

During different seasons, I save my cleaned vegetable trimmings. I place them in a bag in my freezer. When the bag is full, I add a few herbs and water to the veggies. That combination simmers into a delicious veggie broth. For pennies I replace expensive veggie bouillon cubes and chicken broth.

Bulk buying has helped us save a great deal on our monthly budget. As important as the money savings is the time savings. Everything but produce is purchased in bulk. Long-storing veggies, such as carrots, onions, etc., can also be bought in bulk. This form of buying saves me many trips to the grocery store throughout the month. We all know that we can go into a store for one thing and come out with five items. Reducing my trips to the store saves money and also time.

A well-stocked pantry allows me to have what I need to make nearly any meal that we want. To maintain a well-stocked pantry, I keep a running grocery list. As we come close to running out of an item, it immediately goes on the list by category. Those categories include store, co-op (my food-buying club), and other. When I go to the store, I already have a prepared list of needed items.

I can remember prices fairly easily. If I see a food item on sale at the store that is on my co-op list, and that sale price is better, I buy it. Keeping my eyes open and my lists handy has saved us hundreds, if not thousands, of dollars over the years.

How many of you have looked for recipes in magazines or cookbooks? For years I pored over cookbooks and tried recipe after recipe. Yes, we had some great meals, but the time requirement was extensive. I became discouraged and reverted to our basic tried-and-true dishes. This produced boredom. Then we would eat out: That was too expensive.

When we decided to change our diet, the thought of meal planning became overwhelming. Now I had fewer books, fewer skills, and less experience. What could I do? What I have learned over the years in the area of meal planning can save you the torment of that situation.

Out of sheer frustration, I tackled the problem. Nearly a year ago, I devised an entirely different method of meal planning. It is so simple anyone can use it. Variation is a built-in byproduct of this method, as are produce seasonality and individual preferences. What could be easier?

Traditional menu planning requires making a menu for each meal for each day of the week. Selecting seven breakfast, seven lunch, and seven dinner menus (for a total of twenty-one menus) per week is truly overwhelming! Over fifty years, that is 54,600 menus. That could easily cause depression to waltz in. Menu planning had become too complicated for me. I had to find a way to simplify that whole process.

Instead of twenty-one menus per week, I selected seven methods of cooking. Into those seven methods, I put the seasonal produce. By having the necessary ingredients on hand, I can decide to cook the meal whenever I want. This method of meal planning allows me to have everything I need to prepare several meals whenever I want. Once again, meals are fun and varied. Many benefits arise from this meal-planning technique. I use and enjoy all of my kitchen gadgets. We eat seasonally and within our budget. Food variety occurs each day. We make smarter food choices without food becoming a legal hassle. Cooking becomes a matter of a few cooking methods instead of a major administrative chore. Let's look at how this process works.

BREAKFASTS

Since breakfast falls in the elimination period of our body clock, our breakfasts are very simple. We primarily eat fresh fruit or have fruit smoothies. Smoothies combine fresh, seasonal fruits; fruit juice; a frozen fruit; and other nutritional additions.

Apple juice is frequently used. However, fresh pineapple, orange, strawberry, guava, and raspberry are other favorite options. Frozen bananas add richness and smoothness. They turn simple fruit juices into the illusion of "ice-cream shakes." Frozen strawberries and other frozen berries or frozen peaches work well, also.

Besides the fruit, we often add sunflower seeds, sesame seeds (very high in calcium), some form of lecithin, and a "green powder." "Green powders," such as KyoGreen (our favorite), contain dried, concentrated juices from grasses and grains. They provide excellent sources of chlorophyll, amino acids, vitamin A, beta-carotene, iron, calcium, and potassium. These "green powders" produce powerful blood builders, free radical scavengers, and an improved immune system. What a way to start each morning!

Having both been raised on "big, hot, heavy breakfasts," Forest and I were pleasantly surprised to find that we had more energy on this type of simple breakfast. Not spending energy digesting a heavy breakfast releases a tremendous amount of energy to us during our morning hours.

Eating a simple breakfast of fruits and/or fruit smoothies makes breakfast meals easy to plan. I simply ensure that I buy lots of fruit and juice. I keep the seeds and other "healthy additives" well stocked in our pantry.

At midmorning we often take a grain break. That is a good time for a muffin, whole-grain cereal, or some hearty pancakes. The ingredients for each of these are kept in my pantry. If you keep a well-stocked pantry, as indicated in chapter 9, you should always have the necessary ingredients to make these items.

I make muffins, pancakes, etc., on the weekends. I always make extra. The extras are frozen for use during the week. When our daughter wants pancakes, she pops the frozen (homemade, whole-grain) pancakes into the toaster. Soon, she has a hot, satisfying grain dish. These homemade versions are cheaper, tastier, and more nutritious than their frozen, commercial counterparts.

LUNCHES

Lunch is another easy meal. Our lunches are composed of one of two things: salads or leftovers. We work at eating as many salads as possible. Having a salad at lunch ensures we are getting our quota of raw veggies.

When salads are too much (we have those days, too), we clean up leftovers. I plan my leftovers. Planned leftovers are a great time and money saver. In my *Meals in 30 Minutes* cookbook, I dedicate an entire chapter to planning leftovers. It details which foods lend themselves to leftovers and creative ways to use those extra foods.

Shopping for lunches means buying plenty of salad fixings. Extra produce is always kept on hand. Special salad ingredients such as artichoke hearts, slivered almonds, dried fruits, cooked beans, etc., are added to our salads for variety. Our salads are new and different each day.

DINNERS

Dinners provide the opportunity for using our seven cooking methods. Here is where the fun begins. Using the different cooking methods immediately adds variety and creativity to your evening meals.

As I show you a sample week, remember, you choose the cooking methods. The methods we enjoy may not work for your family. You may not even know seven different methods of cooking. This is an opportunity to stretch your culinary talents. It will open a new dimension of meal preparation to you.

Even if I set Monday as stir-fry night, you can always decide to make Monday a soup night. The method and its assigned day are totally up to you. You pick the cooking method and you assign the day. Here is one of our sample weeks:

Monday	Stir-fry
Tuesday	Soup or main-dish salad
Wednesday	Steamed or baked vegetables (meat is an optional addition)
Thursday	Pasta or cooked grains
Friday	Crockpot or casserole
Saturday	Ethnic dishes
Sunday	Forest cooks, leftovers, or dine out (one of my favorite nights)

Let's take a look at how this format works in a little more detail. Once I have learned which vegetables are in season and on sale, I select the veggies for the week. I try to include ten to fifteen different veggies for the week. That may sound like a lot to you. However, when you count onions, garlic, celery, carrots, and several kinds of lettuce, you are already up to six or seven items. These veggies will constitute the basis of our dinner menus.

For example, several of those veggies can go into Monday's stir-fry. Many recipes exist for stir-fry sauces. Serve a stir-fry (with or without meat) over cooked brown rice. This is a low-fat, delicious meal. Since you will only do a stir-fry weekly, try varying the vegetables, sauces, and grain. Many excellent cookbooks have recipes for stir-fries. Be sure to not overcook the vegetables. If you must err, err closer to too raw than overcooked.

Tuesdays are an easy night, too. A hearty soup or salad can usually be made ahead of time or in a Crockpot. We enjoy black-bean soup with cornbread. The leftover soup is used to make refried beans for burritos later in the week. An example of a hearty salad might be a taco salad (with or without meat, with lots of lettuce). Our daughter especially likes this dish.

Wednesdays are one of our favorite nights. Often we do a baked potato with all kinds of toppings. Sometimes we have other steamed vegetables and maybe a homemade muffin. Toppings range from fat-free sour cream (or a tofu substitute) to chopped green onions to salsa to a few sprouts to a little canola oil and canola seeds. These are only a few of our continually changing options.

We vary the potatoes. From white potatoes to russets to yams to sweet potatoes, we have many options. During the fall and winter we select from the many varieties of winter squash. A variety of other veggies and a hot muffin make a very satisfying meal.

If you want to add meat, add a piece of broiled, baked, or lightly sautéed meat or fish with the veggies. For better food combining, use nonstarchy veggies on a meat night.

With a pasta machine, homemade pasta is a snap to prepare for Thursday. When I make pasta, I make several batches and freeze the extra. When Thursday rolls around, I pull out the pasta, make a simple sauce, add a salad, and another simple meal is ready.

Sometimes I alternate pasta with a cooked grain. One of our favorites is fried rice. We don't actually fry the brown rice, nor do we use eggs. Tamari, veggies, and rice make an excellent fried rice. Any grain can substitute for the brown rice to add variety.

Friday usually takes advantage of a Crockpot or the time-bake setting on my oven. Taking leftover veggies, I build a shepherd's pie (veggie pie with mashed potatoes) or a veggie casserole. This is a good time to make a hearty stew in the Crockpot. Add some homemade bread or another salad, and dinner is ready.

A favorite meal to share with friends is our ethnic meal on

Saturday. Homemade tacos, pizza, or Mexican food easily multiply for others. A pizza stone turns ordinary pizza into a true taste sensation. We make veggie pizzas, Mexican pizzas, salad pizzas, dessert pizzas, and many more varieties. Pizza is simply some type of crust and toppings—which are not limited to pepperoni and sausage, by the way. Expand your horizons and try any of the aforementioned pizzas. You will be pleasantly surprised at how tasty they are.

Forest has committed to handling our Sunday dinner meals. He either takes us out, or he prepares a simple meal at home. Sometimes we go to friends' homes, or we catch up on leftovers from the week. This is a relaxed, easy day and our eating reflects it.

As the months go by, the vegetables and fruits will change with the seasons. We now have dishes we look forward to throughout the year. In the spring we enjoy stewed artichokes. This is a hearty stew of whole artichokes, carrots, potatoes, and a gravy. It is reminiscent of a pot roast (without the roast).

Just as we start to tire of this dish, summer comes and we move into fresh fruit salads. We grill yummy veggie kabobs (marinated with fresh lemon juice, basil, garlic, and a small amount of olive oil) and serve them over homemade pasta.

As melons and other summer produce grows old, we move into autumn. Then we have stuffed squash. Butternut squash is filled with a tasty wild-rice stuffing and lightly covered with a mushroom sauce.

Winter moves us into hearty soups, stews, and casseroles— perfect for nippy nights. Whenever possible, I make a double batch of the evening's meal and freeze it for future use.

How can a person tire of such delicious variety? It really helps to know when different fruits and veggies are in season. Knowing appropriate cooking methods takes advantage of the unique flavor of produce.

It also helps to be familiar with recipes. One tape in our Lifestyle for Health Seminar Series highlights many of our favorite recipes. So often we don't know where to start with a new cookbook. The recipes I highlight work well for families just beginning to change their food choices, as well as for health pros.

SNACKS, DESSERTS, FEASTS

Yes, we eat all of the above. Having healthy snacks handy is very important. I set out a huge fruit bowl in our kitchen. As much as possible, we eat our snacks from that bowl. Because I am willing to spend "snack money" on fruit, we have an abundant variety. Melons, grapes, mangoes, kiwi, and pears, among many other fruits, join the regular apples, oranges, and bananas.

Besides fruit, I make whole-grain baked chips available. Dunking a few chips into a fresh salsa helps satisfy a crunchie craving. Rice cakes with almond butter add protein and energy. Healthy, low-fat granola and trail mixes are also kept handy. Many other healthy snacks are available. Enjoy them and they will replace the old fat-loaded, sugary snacks of yesterday.

As America has flirted with low-fat diets in the past few years, statistics show a significant increase in the consumption of desserts. Most of those desserts have a high fat and sugar content. Additionally, they often rely on processed foods, additives, and other chemicals.

Many people choose to start their food changes with desserts. As they discover the new world of "healthier" desserts, they open themselves to change. Tasty, whole-grain, sugar-free desserts catch their attention. They begin to think, *Maybe healthy food really is a viable option.*

Most people are committed to desserts being in their food selection. Instead of fighting that desire, work with it. Find recipes for healthier desserts. Again, the key is moderation. Too many deserts, even healthier ones, are not good. Learn to use good judgment with your healthier desserts.

Holidays, birthdays, and celebrations are times for feasting. Every culture has its feast days. However, as societies or persons grow in wealth, they often make their regular food intake a diet of "feast" foods. This is the situation in North America. Our daily diet consists of nothing but "feasts."

Celebrations happen, but not every day. Special foods eaten only during special occasions keep those foods special. Let feast foods be for feasting. Take them out of the realm of the ordinary and elevate them into special foods.

We have special foods for Thanksgiving, Christmas, and birthdays. We look forward to them. We enjoy them more because they truly are treats instead of the normal, daily fare. As the years go by, our special foods get simpler. Our tastes change, and so do our feasting choices.

If there are certain foods that you are reluctant to give up, delegate them to the category of feast foods. When a time of celebration (a real celebration, not a craving!) arises, enjoy that food. Be sure it is clean (as free of chemicals as possible).

GROCERY SHOPPING

I combine the seasonal food list with the weekly newspaper specials to determine the produce that I will buy for the week. I include fruit for breakfast, salad fixings for lunch, and the necessary produce for dinner. I add that produce list to the grocery list I keep throughout the week.

As I prepare my store list, I divide the items into categories: produce, grocery (packaged items), meat (if applicable), frozen, bulk/repack, dairy, and bakery. The categories I select are based on the store layout. This organized list speeds me through the store.

I purchase our cleaning, laundry, and food supplements from a local distributor. She delivers these items to our home as I order them. I purchase paper products (toilet paper, paper towels, etc.) quarterly, when they are on sale. With a little advanced planning, grocery shopping has been greatly simplified at the Townsley home!

FASTING

Another form of meal planning at our house is fasting. We regularly fast and have experienced many significant benefits. I do, however, recommend that you work with a qualified professional to supervise any fast. I am not giving you a prescription. I am sharing my experiences.

I have fasted in many ways for many reasons. When I first began to work with our nutritionist, I fasted to remove toxins and identify food allergies. That fast started with a juice fast and progressed to fruits and vegetables. Foods were reintroduced one at a time to identify any reaction, allergy, or sensitivity. This is often called an elimination diet or fast.

Later, I experienced a gallbladder attack and passed several stones. The pain of this experience is quite significant and causes many people to opt for surgery. I chose not to take the surgical route. After consulting with our nutritionist, I selected a "fast" route (no pun intended). I went on another supervised fast, dumping many toxins and passing about thirty to forty stones (in a much less painful manner). I consulted a physician for an ultrasound and received a clean bill of health. The results of the ultrasound showed a clean gallbladder with *no* stones, much to the doctor's surprise.

Many people confuse fasting with starvation. Much of this misunderstanding comes from the medical community, where the terms are interchangeable. Unfortunately, this is founded more on prejudice than on truth. Fasting is one way to:

▶ remain in good health
▶ reduce pain and dis-ease
▶ control weight
▶ prolong life

Fasting is the abstinence from all food or a particular food(s). Fasting is a normal biological process in the body. A natural loss of appetite during illness is the body's way of saying, "I don't want food. I want to heal and regenerate." This is a form of fasting that everybody has experienced at one time or another. Take advantage of these times. Let the body rest, restore itself, and cleanse itself. Our body will tell us when we need food.

I am aware of at least thirteen types of fasts. We will look at only a few of those forms of fasting.

Absolute fast. This entails abstinence from all food and liquid except pure water. In this fast, hunger leaves after two or three days and will return when the fast should be stopped.

Partial fast. This fast refrains from certain types of food. One that works well for detoxification is abstaining from all foods except raw vegetables, fruits, nuts, and seeds.

Juice fast. In this fast, all solid food is eliminated. Only fresh fruit and/or vegetable juices are taken. This is an effective cleansing fast. It is often done for therapeutic reasons.

Liquid fast. Any liquid—and only liquid—may be consumed in this fast, including broth, juice, water, etc. It is not considered the best fast for cleansing. However, it is convenient for spiritual reasons and/or weight control.

We have done all of the above forms of fasting. We now fast weekly. Our appetites are beginning to surrender control to that discipline. Fasting increases our mental alertness, our ability to stay focused, and our discipline. It also serves as a mild cleanse. Again, I recommend that you work with a health-care provider when considering any form of fasting.

Tonight is just a normal night for us. We are neither fasting nor feasting. We are nourishing our bodies with an ordinary meal. The house is in order, the table is set, and a delicious, low-fat vegetarian lasagna (with homemade noodles) is heating in the oven. A salad chills in the refrigerator, while veggies steam in the steamer. It's time to join together as a family and enjoy a nutritious, tasty meal. We close another day on our road to health.

Now it is your turn. You know enough to make you and your family healthier. However, that knowledge must be applied. Take your new smarts and make smart food choices. A clean bill of health is one of the most valuable tests you will ever pass!

Good health (mental, emotional, physical, and spiritual) puts us in an optimal position to live our lives with purpose and fulfillment. Learn what you can, and apply what you know. You will become a person alive to your purpose in life.

Cleanses

C leansing the body is similar to cleaning house. Just as dusting requires a different process from vacuuming, so a liver cleanse requires a different process from a colon cleanse. The following cleansing suggestions are just that: suggestions. *No cleanse should be implemented without the supervision of a health-care provider. These suggestions are not meant to be prescriptions.*

Today's environment and our overall culture make it difficult for the eliminative organs (colon, skin, kidneys, lungs, and liver) to function normally. Each of these organs can benefit from annual cleansing. Failing to periodically cleanse these organs causes toxic build-up, which eventually can produce a health crisis of some kind.

The most common organs to cleanse are the colon (large intestine), liver, gallbladder, lungs, kidneys, and the skin. Suggested cleanses for each organ follow.

Colon (Large Intestine) Cleansing
Poor diet (that is, white bread, cakes, cookies, meat, dairy products, pasta, and overcooked veggies), antibiotics, stress, and lack of water take a heavy toll on the colon. Since this is the primary

organ for elimination, colon toxicity creates a major problem for the body.

▶ Enemas and/or colonics help stimulate the peristaltic activity of the muscles found in the large intestine. A colonic is a continuous enema, usually administered by a professional. A colema is a combined enema-colonic that can be self-administered at home. The best source of information on enemas, colonics, and colemas can be found in the following book:

Tissue Cleansing Through Bowel Management by Bernard Jensen, D.C., Nutritionist (Bernard Jensen Enterprises, 24360 Old Wagon Road, Escondido, CA 92027)

▶ "Exercising" helps strengthen the colon muscles. Ann Wigmore, in her book *The Hippocrates Diet and Health Program*, suggests the abdominal lift: "To do this, bend over slightly, placing your hands just above your knees. Blow all the air out of your lungs, forcibly, and hold it out. A natural vacuum will be created, and with it, suck up your abdomen, pulling the stomach muscles in. Relax without inhaling, to push the stomach out. While holding your breath, try to make your stomach as large and round as possible. This movement should be performed ten times. Stand, breathe slowly and deeply." Perform three or four sets of these exercises (ten repeats in each set).

People who have sedentary jobs often have a dropped colon. Exercising on a slant board can take advantage of gravitational pull to help reposition the colon into its correct position. Work with a health-care provider to determine the type and number of exercises to do on a slant board. One of the better ones is bicycle pedaling, while lying head down on the slant board.

A tennis ball or small rubber ball can also be used to massage the colon. Rub the ball around in a circle over the abdominal area. The round surface of the ball gets down into the bowel area and is similar to internal exercising.

▶ Bentonite and psyllium powder are often used for intestinal cleansing. (Suggested brands include Veico 77, VIT-RA-

TOX 16 and 19, Sonne 7, and Nature's Sunshine.) Use a jar with a tight cover. Put one-half to one inch of fruit juice, eight ounces of purified water, one or two tablespoons of bentonite, and a heaping teaspoon of psyllium powder into the jar. Place the lid on tightly. Shake vigorously for ten to fifteen seconds, or until the mixture is well blended, and then drink it. Evacuations may not occur until the second day, thereby causing a temporary feeling of fullness. Unusual eliminated fecal matter is a result of the colon's toxic waste, not the cleansing solution. This process can be done once or twice a day during the cleansing time.

▶ During watermelon season, watermelon can be used for a good cleanse. Consuming watermelon for three to five days cleanses the kidneys and colon. The extra fluids help pick up and remove colonic debris.

▶ Fasting one day a week (juice diet or fruit and *rest*) is helpful in resting the body and speeding the process of eliminating toxic materials.

▶ After colon cleansing, maintenance is important. Eating a diet rich in fiber from raw veggies and fruit is very helpful. Some of the suggested supplements include zinc; vitamins E, C, and A; brewer's yeast; blackstrap molasses; and lecithin. Vitamin A is reputed to be good for bowel disturbances, ulcerations, colitis, and fighting infections. Brewer's yeast provides B vitamins. Cider vinegar (preferably raw) is also helpful in balancing the bowel environment.

Liver and Gallbladder Cleansing
The liver is the major organ for detoxification. It affects the overall health of the other organs and the blood. The liver stores and processes many nutrients, pollutants, and waste materials. Fried foods, hydrogenated fats, rancid oils, chemical additives, tobacco, alcohol, and environmental pollutants weaken the liver. Bile, stored in the gallbladder, is the carrier for liver wastes, including excess cholesterol. Bile also helps in the assimilation of fats and in digestion. With a poor diet, bile will produce solid particles called gallstones. A weakened, congested liver will manifest itself through skin problems, poor

eyesight, hair loss, and hemorrhoids.

▶ Green drinks, such as KyoGreen, are rich in minerals and chlorophyll and help cleanse the liver. Lemon juice in warm water helps cleanse and works as an antiseptic agent. Fresh carrot juice, high in pro-vitamin A, helps stimulate the flow of bile. Beet juice (be sure to dilute it with another juice) helps stimulate the gallbladder, liver, and kidneys.

▶ The traditional olive-oil cleanse is a more serious cleanse. Using this cleanse, under the care of my nutritionist, helped me to pass over fifty gallstones. I use this cleanse once a year. Be sure to be under the supervision of a health-care provider. Five days prior to the cleanse, consume as much apple juice (preferably fresh or unpasteurized) as possible. As much as one gallon of juice per day is recommended. The juice may be consumed as a juice fast or with light meals.

On the sixth day, after lunch, dissolve one to two tablespoons of Epsom salt in three ounces of warm, distilled water. Drink this mixture. It may be followed with a little citrus juice, preferably fresh.

Four hours after lunch, take an enema. Try to retain the enema for up to fifteen minutes. Coffee enemas are best. Bring two tablespoons of coffee and two cups of water to a boil. Let stand fifteen minutes before using. Strain and use in the enema bag. Five hours after lunch, repeat the Epsom salt drink.

At bedtime, drink one-half cup of unrefined oil followed by citrus juice (the citrus juice can be mixed with the olive oil). Immediately upon finishing the oil, go to bed and lie on the right side with the right knee drawn up toward the chin for thirty minutes. This encourages the oil to drain from the stomach and helps contents from the gallbladder and liver move into the small intestine. Elimination from this cleanse should occur the following day, usually in the afternoon.

▶ Liver packs can help the liver drain and cleanse itself. To do a liver pack, soak a cotton cloth (for example, a washcloth) with castor oil. Place the cloth over the liver (under the right rib cage) and cover with a plastic wrap. Place a cloth or towel that has been immersed in hot water (squeeze out excess water) over the plastic wrap. Cover with another layer of plastic wrap. Place a hot-water bottle (preferably) or heating pad over all layers. Rest with this pack over the liver for ninety minutes. Do this for three days and then refrain from the procedure for four days. This may be repeated several times.

I have found this procedure helps drain the liver. Greenish stools (bowel movements) may occur after the cleanse. Some people find they have more energy after the packs.

▶ Many commercial cleansing programs are available in health-food stores. Bioforce has a good "spring cleaning" program designed to eliminate toxins. Follow the manufacturer's directions for best results.

Lung Cleansing

Breathing is the body's way of exchanging gases in the lungs. The blood is cleansed of carbon dioxide and other waste products. Oxygenated air is breathed in, absorbed by the blood, and delivered throughout the body. A diet heavy with dairy, white flour, and pasta, along with smoking and air pollution, causes excessive accumulations of mucus in the sinuses and bronchial tubes. This mucus affects the lungs and all of the other eliminatory organs (skin, kidneys, liver, and colon).

▶ Eating foods low, or lacking, in mucus is one of the best ways to cleanse the lungs. Moderate uses of foods such as raw green onions, garlic, and fresh ginger help reduce mucus. Chlorophyll has been known to increase the red blood cell count, thereby helping the body carry more oxygen.

▶ Breathing exercises are another way to cleanse the lungs. Most adults use only 25 percent of their lung capacity. Deep breathing should begin in the stomach, which will then push out the diaphragm. Inhale deeply, then release the air slowly. Do this often throughout the day.

Kidney Cleansing

Each day, 4,000 quarts of blood flow through our kidneys. There, the blood is cleansed of its waste, so that the acid-alkaline balance of the blood can be maintained. Body temperature is also regulated by the kidneys. The kidneys eliminate drugs, pollutants, and bacterial waste from the body. With our current lifestyle and environment, the kidneys are one of the most stressed organs. Polluted air, water, food, drugs, and other pollutants put heavy stress on the kidneys.

▶ To first cleanse the kidneys, eliminate refined foods, salt, meat, caffeine, alcohol, tobacco, and impure water.

▶ Green drinks, such as KyoGreen, help to cleanse the kidneys.

▶ Watermelon juice works as an effective diuretic. The rind, seeds, and pulp can all be put into the juicer. Watermelon juice helps to reverse fluid retention.

▶ Beet juice helps to tone the kidneys. Lemon juice is a mild diuretic. Sea vegetables are rich in minerals necessary for detoxification. If possible, use several different sea vegetables in your diet. Using them in soups or when cooking beans is an easy way to add them to your diet. Kelp powder and other sea vegetables are added to many condiments.

Skin Cleansing

The largest organ is the skin. Nearly five pounds of waste material leave the skin each day. The kidneys, lungs, and colon remove about two pounds. Clogged pores in the skin place an extra burden on these other eliminatory organs. Skin blemishes indicate that the body is toxic. Complete body cleansing will usually cause these blemishes to disappear.

Every twenty-seven days, we have an entirely new skin surface. This shedding takes place one cell at a time. Overly dry skin clogs the skin and prevents it from effectively doing its elimination.

▶ Skin brushing is one of the most effective ways to cleanse the skin. Skin brushing will also help stimulate the lymphatic system. This system helps remove toxins throughout the body. Skin brushing is basically a "dry" bath. With a nonnylon, natural-bristle brush, brush the body vigorously for about five minutes each morning before showering. Brush in circles working toward the heart. Skin brushing removes the uric acid crystals and other acid wastes from the pores of the skin. Follow this dry brushing with a shower and the use of a loofah sponge. This will wash off the loosened dry skin.

▶ Use gentle soaps on the body. Avoid detergents and strong deodorant soaps. Liquid soaps rinse more easily. Excess soaping removes valuable skin oils, necessary for skin lubrication.

▶ Alternate warm and cold water at the end of your shower. This process stimulates the pores in the skin.

▶ Therapeutic massage is another excellent way to cleanse the skin and the body. Therapeutic massage is different from simple massage in that the therapist is knowledgeable of the body and the various ways to stimulate the organs. Mineral oil should be avoided when massaging. Simple oils, such as olive, almond, and coconut, are fine to use for massage.

Cleansing Baths

There is a long history of the use of cleansing baths in Germany and in the naturopathic community. These baths are quite effective in the removal of environmental toxins, heavy metal deposits, and radiation, which in this period of history represent a frequently encountered low-grade and continuous drain on the immune system and on general body functioning.

Almost all of us have unknowingly accumulated our fair share of heavy metal deposits in our tissues. Because of nuclear fallout, radioactive proliferation, toxic dumps, etc., you may appear symptom-free, but in actuality carry within you "a silent time bomb." If you have experienced numerous x-rays, surgery, or CAT scans, worked before computer terminals or with chemicals and fumes (e.g. photocopy equipment, printing presses, automobiles, street fumes), you can assume that you have a fair share of toxic "gunk" in your body. Taking a series of cleansing baths is an inexpensive and pleasant way to ensure the maintenance of your health.

Because baths can sometimes be experienced as temporarily draining, they are best taken before bedtime. Drinking extra fluids is recommended, especially if you sweat a lot after bathing. If you are in a state of ill health or of weakened constitution, it is advised to replenish beneficial minerals that may have leached out through the bathing process by consuming seaweed or vegetables high in minerals, such as leafy greens, zucchini, parsley, green beans, or jicama on the day following the bath.

Feeling uncomfortable, irritable, or edgy after bathing is frequently the result of toxins being pulled out of the body and is a sign that the baths are working for you.

When taking cleansing baths, fill the bath to the top (duct tape can be used to close off the overflow) of the tub. Immerse everything except your face and hair. If you get uncomfortable or dizzy while bathing, sit up for a while before returning to a reclining position. Do not lengthen the recommended time for bathing. Experiment until you find the right warm temperature, which is most conducive to pleasant bathing for you.[1]

Sample Cleansing Baths
   2 to 4 pounds Epsom salt
   1 cup raw apple-cider vinegar
   1 tablespoon dry ginger
   1 tablespoon (or less) cayenne pepper
   Warm, not hot, water

Soak up to half an hour. The cayenne pepper does produce gases that can cause a slight burning sensation. Space these baths a week apart.

   Juice of 2 to 3 lemons
   Hot water

Soak up to fifteen minutes. Average of six baths, one week apart.

   2 pounds sea salt and 2 pounds baking soda
   Hot water

Soak for twenty to thirty minutes.

Fasting
Regular fasting is one of the easiest ways to cleanse the body. As food is eaten, it must be masticated (chewed), digested, assim-

ilated, and then the waste is eliminated. It takes a tremendous amount of energy for the body to process that food through the thirty-foot tube that goes from the mouth to the rectum. It takes even more energy for the body to pump blood, pass liquid through the kidneys, and breathe in oxygen. Fasting gives the body a period of rest from the food process.

When we stop eating, we transfer all of the energy used to process food into eliminating body toxins. Fasting one day a week (for twenty-four to thirty-six hours) totals fifty-two days a year of cleansing the body. Those fifty-two days become days of rest—cleansing restoration for the body, mind, and soul. Needless to say, it also saves money.

Fasts are not meant to "cure" diseases. The body is designed to cure itself, when it is in its optimal condition. Fasting helps the body strengthen itself so that it can do the job it has been designed to do. As Paul Bragg says in *The Miracle of Fasting*, "Fasting is the key which unlocks Nature's storehouse of energy. . . . It is a personal duty that only YOU can perform."[2]

Fasting will help reduce the acidity of the body, which is caused by a diet heavy in sugar, sugar products, coffee, tea, alcohol, meats, fish, and grains. To help the fasting process, increase the amounts of alkaline foods, which include fruits, vegetables, seeds, and nuts. *If you choose to fast while you have a disease, be under the strict supervision of a health-care provider.*

Many fasting experts recommend only the consumption of distilled water while fasting. Some nutritionists will allow fresh fruit or vegetable juices. Check with your health-care provider to ensure which type of fasting is best for you. A person who regularly fasts each week and has completed four to six fasts of three to four days each is probably ready for a more extended fast. After at least six months of this process, enough toxins should have been released to allow a person to easily handle a seven-day fast. Continuing this process would prepare a person for a ten-day, twenty-one day, and possibly a forty-day fast. Many short (twenty-four to thirty-six hour) fasts with a regular lifestyle of quality food, exercise, and rest can do as much as one extended fast.

The day prior to fasting, it is best to consume raw salads, fresh fruits, and at least seven to eight glasses of pure water. When doing an absolute fast (distilled water only), a teaspoon of fresh lemon juice and one-third teaspoon of raw honey can be added to each glass of water. This will help remove mucus and toxins from the body. Be sure to drink as much water as possible during a fast.

Following a fast, the first food you eat should be raw vegetables. This roughage will help sweep the colon of loosened debris. Follow the raw vegetables with one or two cooked vegetables. The worst foods to eat following a fast are meat, dairy products, fish, nuts, seeds, or sugar.

Mail-Order Information

Food Items

Albert's Organics
Los Angeles, CA 90058
(213)234-4595

Colvado Date Co.
51-352 Hwy 86
P.O. Box 98
Coachella, CA 92236
(619)398-3441

Erneston Organic Produce
West Palm Beach, FL
(407)832-2446

Glasser Farms Fruits
Miami, FL
(305)238-7747

Hardscrabble Enterprises
Route 6 Box 42
Cherry Grove, WV 26804
(304)567-2727

Kahulla Gardens
P.O. Box 2328
Borrego Springs, CA 92004
(619)540-5693

Mountain Ark Trading Co.
Fayetteville, AR 72701
(800)643-8909

Sprout Delights, Inc.
Essene Bread
Miami, FL 33168
(303)687-5880

Food Items (continued)

UniTea Herbs
1919 D 19th St.
Boulder, CO 80302
(303)443-1248

Walnut Acres Natural Foods
Penns Creek, PA 17862
(717)837-0601

Seeds

Cross Seed Company
HC 69 Box 2
Bunker Hill, KS 67626
(913)483-6163

Jaffe Brothers
P.O. Box 636
Valley Center, CA 92082
(619)749-1133

Diamond K Enterprises
RR 1 Box 30
St. Charles, MN 55952
(507)932-4308

Living Farms
P.O. Box 50
Tracy, MN 56175
(507)629-4431

Equipment

Bee Beyer's Food Dryers
1154 Roberta Lane
Los Angeles, CA
(213)472-8961

Lifestyle for Health
7302 South Eudora Way
Littleton, CO 80122
(303)771-9357

Cuisinart Processors
Greenwich, CT 06830
(203)975-4600

Oster Blenders
Professional Products
Route 9 Box 541
McMinnville, TN 37110
(615)668-4121

Excalibur
6083 Power Inn Road
Sacramento, CA 95824
(916)381-4254

Water-Purification Systems

Best Water Systems
Local Shaklee Representative
Water Factory Systems
68 Fairbanks
Irvine, CA 92718
(800)767-5511

WHOLESALERS

If you are unable to buy health food in your local stores, the following information can help you work with the wholesalers in your area. Possibilities include food-buying clubs, co-ops, and direct buying.

For further information on computerized ordering services for co-op services, contact:

Co-op Services
P.O. Box 364
Franklin, IN 46131
(800)685-8886

Wholesalers by State

Alabama

Arnie Wolman Co., Inc.
Cornucopia Natural Foods
H-P Distributors
International Specialty
  Supply
Mountain People's
  Warehouse

Orange Blossom Coop
  Warehouse
Ozark Cooperative
  Warehouse
Tree of Life Midwest
Tree of Life Southeast
Vitality Distributors, Inc.

Alaska

Arnie Wolman Co., Inc.
Northbest Natural
  Products
Nutra Source

Ray's Food Services, Inc.
Tree of Life Northwest
Tree of Life West

Arizona

Arnie Wolman Co., Inc.
Falcon Trading Co.
Food for Health Co.
Fruit of the Land
Koster

Mountain People's
  Warehouse
Nature's Best
Tree of Life/Southwest Div.
Tucson Co-op Warehouse

Arkansas

Arnie Wolman Co., Inc.
H-P Distributors
Koster

Ozark Cooperative
    Warehouse
Tree of Life/Southwest Div.

California

Almil Nutritional
    Products, Inc.
Arnie Wolman Co., Inc.
Cedarland Foods Co.
Clarity Distributing
Falcon Trading Co.
Food for Health Co.
Fowler Bros. Distr.
    Natrl. Fd.
Fruit of the Land
Glorybee Foods
Health Run

Koster
Maranatha Natural Foods
Mountain People's
    Warehouse
Natural Foods Northwest
Nature's Best
Northbest Natural Products
North Coast Foods
Quong Hop & Co.
Ray's Food Services, Inc.
Tucson Co-op Warehouse

Colorado

Arnie Wolman Co., Inc.
Falcon Trading Co.
Food for Health Co.
Mountain People's
    Warehouse

Nature's Best
Rainbow Distributing, Inc.
Tree of Life/Southwest Div.
Tucson Co-op Warehouse

Connecticut

A.C.D. Sales Co.
All Natural Distributors, Inc.
Arnie Wolman Co., Inc.
Cornucopia Natural Foods
F & D Distributors
Forcite Distributing
Garden Spot Distributors

Gold Coast Traders, Inc.
Neshaminy Valley
    Natural Foods
Northeast Cooperatives
Stow Mills
Tree of Life, Northeast

Delaware

Arnie Wolman Co., Inc.
Cornucopia Natural
  Foods
Garden Spot Distributors
Genesee Natural Foods, Inc.
Neshaminy Valley Natural
  Foods
Stow Mills
Tree of Life, Northeast
Tree of Life Southeast

District of Columbia

Arnie Wolman Co., Inc.
Cornucopia Natural Foods
Federation-Ohio River
  Co-ops
Frankferd Farms Foods
Garden Spot Distributors
Neshaminy Valley Natural
  Foods
Stow Mills
Tree of Life, Northeast
Tree of Life Southeast

Florida

Arnie Wolman Co., Inc.
Cornucopia Natural Foods
Forcite Distributing
Health Foods, Inc.
H-P Distributors
Orange Blossom Coop
  Warehouse
Sun Ray Products
  Distribution
Tree of Life Southeast
Vitality Distributors, Inc.

Georgia

Arnie Wolman Co., Inc.
Cornucopia Natural Foods
Country Life Natural
  Foods
Health Foods, Inc.
H-P Distributors
International Specialty
  Supply
Orange Blossom Coop
  Warehouse
Ozark Cooperative
  Warehouse
Tree of Life Midwest
Tree of Life Southeast
Vitality Distributors, Inc.

Hawaii

Arnie Wolman Co., Inc.
Cedarlane Foods Co.
Falcon Trading Co.
Fowler Bros. Distr.
  Natrl. Fd.
Koster

Hawaii (continued)

Maui Style Wholesale
  Natural Foods
Mountain People's
  Warehouse
Nature's Best

Nutra Source
Shojin Natural Food, Inc.
Tree of Life Northwest
Tree of Life West

Idaho

Arnie Wolman Co., Inc.
Food for Health Co.
Health Food Distributors,
  Inc.
Mountain People's
  Warehouse

Natural Foods Northwest
Nature's Best
Northbest Natural Products
Nutra Source
Tree of Life Northwest

Illinois

Arnie Wolman Co., Inc.
Blooming Prairie
  Warehouse
Country Life Natural
  Foods
Garden Food Products
Goodness Greeness
Health Food Distributors,
  Inc.

Health Foods, Inc.
North Farm Cooperative
Palko Distributing Company
Rainbow Distributing, Inc.
Speciality Health Foods
Stow Mills
Sunshower Farm
Tree of Life Midwest
U.T.D. Company

Indiana

A. B. Wise & Sons, Inc.
Arnie Wolman Co., Inc.
Blooming Prairie
  Warehouse
Country Life Natural Foods
Federation-Ohio River
  Co-ops
Garden Food Products
Goodness Greeness
Health Foods, Inc.

H-P Distributors
Kramer Food Company
North Farm Cooperative
Palko Distributing Company
Rainbow Distributing, Inc.
Rosewood Products, Inc.
Stow Mills
Sunshower Farm
Tree of Life Midwest
U.T.D. Company

Iowa

Arnie Wolman Co., Inc.
Blooming Prairie Natural
  Foods
Blooming Prairie
  Warehouse
Goodness Greeness
Health Foods, Inc.
Palko Distributing Company
Tree of Life Midwest
U.T.D. Company

Kansas

Arnie Wolman Co., Inc.
Blooming Prairie
  Warehouse
Mountain People's
  Warehouse
Ozark Cooperative Warehouse
Palko Distributing Company
Tree of Life/
  Southwest Div.

Kentucky

A. B. Wise & Sons, Inc.
Arnie Wolman Co., Inc.
Country Life Natural Foods
Federation-Ohio River
  Co-ops
Goodness Greeness
Health Foods, Inc.
H-P Distributors
Palko Distributing Company
Stow Mills
Tree of Life Midwest

Louisiana

Arnie Wolman Co., Inc.
H-P Distributors
Ozark Cooperative
  Warehouse
Tree of Life Southeast
Tree of Life/
  Southwest Div.

Maine

All Natural Distributors,
  Inc.
Associated Buyers
Cornucopia Natural Foods
Forcite Distributing
Northeast Cooperatives
Stow Mills

Maryland

All Natural Distributors,
  Inc.
Cornucopia Natural Foods
Federation-Ohio River
  Co-ops
Frankferd Farms Foods

Maryland (continued)
Garden Spot Distributors P.N.Q.
Genesee Natural Foods, Inc. Stow Mills
Neshaminy Valley Natural Tree of Life, Northeast
   Foods Tree of Life Southeast

Massachusetts
All Natural Distributors, Inc. Gold Coast Traders, Inc.
Arnie Wolman Co., Inc. Neshaminy Valley Natural
Associated Buyers   Foods
Cornucopia Natural Foods Northeast Cooperatives
Forcite Distributing Stow Mills
Garden Spot Distributors Tree of Life, Northeast

Michigan
Blooming Prairie Warehouse Health Foods, Inc.
Common Health Kramer Food Company
   Warehouse North Farm Cooperative
Country Life Natural O-Jib-Wa Vitamin Co.
   Foods Palko Distributing Co.
Federation-Ohio River Rainbow Distributing, Inc.
   Co-ops Rosewood Products, Inc.
Garden Food Products Stow Mill
Goodness Greeness Sunshower Farm
Health Food Distributors, Tree of Life Midwest
   Inc. U.T.D. Company

Minnesota
Blooming Prairie Natural Meadow Farm Foods
   Foods North Farm Cooperative
Common Health Tochi Products
   Warehouse Tree of Life Midwest
Country Life Natural Foods U.T.D. Company
Health Foods, Inc.

Mississippi
H-P Distributors Tree of Life Midwest
Ozark Cooperative Tree of Life Southeast
   Warehouse Tree of Life/Southwest Div.

Missouri

Blooming Prairie
  Warehouse
Country Life Natural
  Foods
Goodness Greeness
Health Foods, Inc.
H-P Distributors
North Farm Cooperative

Ozark Cooperative
  Warehouse
Palko Distributing
  Company
Tree of Life Midwest
Tree of Life/
  Southwest Div.
U.T.D. Company

Montana

Common Health
  Warehouse
Food for Health Co.
Maranatha Natural Foods
Mountain People's
  Warehouse

Nature's Best
Northbest Natural Products
North Farm Cooperative
Nutra Source
Ray's Food Services, Inc.
Tree of Life Northwest

Nebraska

Blooming Prairie
  Warehouse
Country Life Natural
  Foods
Fruit of the Land

Health Foods, Inc.
Health Run
Palko Distributing Company
Tree of Life, Northeast
Tree of Life/Southwest Div.

Nevada

Food for Health Co.
Mountain People's
  Warehouse

Nature's Best
Tucson Co-op Warehouse

New Hampshire

All Natural Distributors, Inc.
Associated Buyers
Cornucopia Natural Foods
Forcite Distributors

Garden Spot Distributors
Northeast Cooperatives
Stow Mills
Tree of Life, Northeast

New Jersey

A.C.D. Sales Co.	Health Waters, Inc.
All Natural Distributors, Inc.	Island Natural, Inc.
Clear Eye Natural Foods	Neshaminy Valley Natural
Cornucopia Natural Foods	Foods
Eat-Rite Dist., Inc.	P.N.Q.
Forcite Distributing	Stow Mills
Garden Spot Distributors	Tree of Life, Northeast
Genesee Natural Foods, Inc.	Tree of Life Southeast
Gold Coast Traders, Inc.	

New Mexico

Falcon Trading Co.	Mountain People's Warehouse
Food for Health Co.	Nature's Best
Fruit of the Land	Tree of Life/Southwest Div.
Koster	Tucson Co-op Warehouse

New York

A.C.D. Sales Co.	Health Waters, Inc.
All Natural Distributors, Inc.	Island Natural, Inc.
Clear Eye Natural Foods	Neshaminy Valley Natural
Cornucopia Natural Foods	Foods
Eat-Rite Dist., Inc.	Northeast Cooperatives
Forcite Distributing	P.N.Q.
Garden Spot Distributors	Stow Mills
Genesee Natural Foods, Inc.	Tree of Life, Northeast
Gold Coast Traders, Inc.	

North Carolina

Cornucopia Natural Foods	Forcite Distributing
Country Life Natural Foods	H-P Distributors
Federation-Ohio River	Tree of Life Southeast
Co-ops	

North Dakota

Common Health Warehouse	Food for Health Co.
Country Life Natural Foods	Health Foods, Inc.

North Dakota (continued)
Meadow Farm Foods
North Farm Cooperative
Tochi Products

Tree of Life Midwest
Tree of Life Northwest

Ohio
A. B. Wise & Sons, Inc.
Clear Eye Natural Foods
Country Life Natural Foods
Federation-Ohio River
   Co-ops
Frankferd Farms Foods
Garden Spot Distributors
Genesee Natural Foods, Inc.
Goodness Greeness
Health Food Distributors,
   Inc.

Health Foods, Inc.
H-P Distributors
Kramer Food Company
North Farm Cooperative
Palko Distributing Company
Rainbow Distributing, Inc.
Rosewood Products, Inc.
Stow Mills
Tree of Life Midwest

Oklahoma
Falcon Trading Co.
Ozark Cooperative
   Warehouse

Tree of Life/
   Southwest Div.

Oregon
Clarity Distributing
Falcon Trading Co.
Fruit of the Land
Glorybee Foods
Maranatha Natural Foods

Mountain People's Warehouse
Northbest Natural Products
Nutra Source
Ray's Food Services, Inc.
Tree of Life Northwest

Pennsylvania
A.C.D. Sales Co.
All Natural Distributors, Inc.
Clear Eye Natural Foods
Cornucopia Natural Foods
Federation-Ohio River
   Co-ops
Forcite Distributing

Frankferd Farms Foods
Garden Spot Distributors
Genesee Natural Foods, Inc.
Goodness Greeness
Health Foods, Inc.
Neshaminy Valley Natural
   Foods

Pennsylvania (continued)
Palko Distributing Co.   Tree of Life, Northeast
P.N.Q.   Tree of Life Midwest
Rosewood Products, Inc.   Tree of Life Southeast
Stow Mills

Rhode Island
All Natural Distributors, Inc. Northeast Cooperatives
Cornucopia Natural Foods   Stow Mills
Forcite Distributing   Tree of Life, Northeast
Garden Spot Distributors
Neshaminy Valley Natural
    Foods

South Carolina
Cornucopia Natural Foods   H-P Distributors
Forcite Distributing   Tree of Life Southeast

South Dakota
Blooming Prairie Natural   Food for Health Co.
    Foods   North Farm Cooperative
Blooming Prairie   Tochi Products
    Warehouse   Tree of Life Midwest
Common Health Warehouse

Tennessee
Cornucopia Natural Foods   Ozark Cooperative
Country Life Natural Foods   Warehouse
Federation-Ohio River   Palko Distributing Company
    Co-ops   Stow Mills
H-P Distributors   Tree of Life Midwest
International Specialty   Tree of Life Southeast
    Supply   Tree of Life/Southwest Div.

Texas
Food for Health Co.   Tree of Life/Southwest Div.
Koster   Tucson Co-op Warehouse
Ozark Cooperative
    Warehouse

Utah

Food for Health Co.
Mountain People's
    Warehouse

Nature's Best
Ray's Food Services, Inc.
Tucson Co-op Warehouse

Vermont

All Natural Distributors, Inc.
Associated Buyers
Cornucopia Natural Foods
Forcite Distributing
Garden Spot Distributors

Neshaminy Valley Natural
    Foods
Northeast Cooperatives
Stow Mills
Tree of Life, Northeast

Virginia

All Natural Distributors, Inc.
Cornucopia Natural Foods
Federation-Ohio River
    Co-ops
Frankferd Farms Foods
Garden Spot Distributors

H-P Distributors
Neshaminy Valley Natural
    Foods
Stow Mills
Tree of Life, Northeast
Tree of Life Southeast

Washington

Clarity Distributing
Fruit of the Land
Glorybee Foods
Mountain People's
    Warehouse

Northbest Natural Products
Nutra Source
Ray's Food Services, Inc.
Tree of Life Northwest

West Virginia

All Natural Distributors, Inc.
Country Life Natural Foods
Federation-Ohio River
    Co-ops

Frankferd Farms Foods
H-P Distributors
Palko Distributing Company
Tree of Life Midwest

Wisconsin

Blooming Prairie
    Natural Foods
Blooming Prairie
    Warehouse

Common Health
    Warehouse
Country Life Natural Foods
Garden Food Products

Wisconsin (continued)
Goodness Greeness
Health Food Distributors, Inc.
Health Foods, Inc.
North Farm Cooperative

Palko Distributing Company
Rainbow Distributing, Inc.
Stow Mills
Tree of Life Midwest
U.T.D. Company

Wyoming
Blooming Prairie Warehouse
Common Health Warehouse
Food for Health Co.

Mountain People's Warehouse
Nature's Best
North Farm Cooperative
Ray's Food Services, Inc.

Wholesaler Addresses
A. B. Wise & Sons, Inc.
4544 Mulhauser Road
Hamilton, OH 45011
(513)874-9642

A.C.D. Sales Co.
35-40 83rd Street
Jackson Heights, NY 11372
(718)335-7293

All Natural Distributors, Inc.
11 Perry Drive
Foxboro, MA 02035
(800)666-2225

Almil Nutritional Products, Inc.
570 West Lambert Road Unit G
Brea, CA 92621
(714)256-1675

Arnie Wolman Co., Inc.
136 SW Washington Street
Corvallis, OR 97333

Associated Buyers
100 Main Street
P.O. Box 207
Somersworth, NH 03878
(603)692-6101

Blooming Prairie Natural Foods
510 Kasota Avenue SE
Minneapolis, MN 55414
(612)378-9774

Blooming Prairie Warehouse
2340 Heinz Road
Iowa City, IA 52240
(319)337-6448

Cedarlane Foods Co.
1864 East 22nd Street
Los Angeles, CA 90058
(800)826-3322

Clarity Distributing
P.O. Box 3516
Santa Rosa, CA 94502
(707)887-2520

Clear Eye Natural Foods
302 Route 89 South
Savannah, NY 13146
(800)724-2233

Common Health Warehouse
1505 North 8th Street
Superior, WI 54880
(715)392-9862

Cornucopia Natural Foods
Div. Oak Haven, Inc.
260 Lake Road
P.O. Box 999
Dayville, CT 06241
(800)433-7395

Country Life Natural Foods
S-3121 Alpine Road
Fountain City, WI 54629
(608)687-8210

Eat-Rite Dist., Inc.
P.O. Box 405
Woodmere, NY 11598
(516)887-FOOD

Falcon Trading Co.
1055—17th Avenue
Santa Cruz, CA 95062
(408)462-1280

F & D Distributors
510 Cornwall Avenue
Cheshire, CT 06410
(203)272-8130

Federation-Ohio River Co-ops
320 East Outerbelt Street
Columbus, OH 43213
(614)861-2446

Food for Health Co.
3655 West Washington Street
Phoenix, AZ 85009
(800)366-1234

Forcite Distributing
256 Garibaldi Avenue
Lodi, NJ 07647
(201)470-5700

Fowler Bros. Distr. Natrl. Fd.
P.O. Box 2324
San Rafael, CA 92912
(415)459-3406

Frankferd Farms Foods
318 Love Road, R.D. #1
Valencia, PA 16059
(412)898-2242

Fruit of the Land
P.O. Box 1913
Newport Beach, CA 92659
(714)644-7755

Garden Food Products
4844 Butterfield Road
Hillside, IL 60162
(708)449-0171

Garden Spot Distributors
438 White Oak Road
New Holland, PA 17447
(800)829-5100

Genesee Natural Foods, Inc.
Route 2 Box 105
Genesee, PA 16923
(814)228-3200

Glorybee Foods
P.O. Box 2744
Eugene, OR 97402
(800)456-7923

Gold Coast Traders, Inc.
3 Pauls Street
Bethel, CT 06801
(800)544-5789

Goodness Greeness
5959 South Lowe
Chicago, IL 60621
(312)224-4411

Health Food Distributors, Inc.
1893 Northwood Drive
Troy, MI 48084
(313)362-4545

Health Foods, Inc.
3949 Commerce Parkway
Miramar, FL 33025
(800)628-2666

Health Foods, Inc.
155 West Higgins Road
Des Plaines, IL 60018
(708)298-8220

Health Run
3403 - 51st Avenue
P.O. Box 231010
Sacramento, CA 95823-0400
(916)421-5037

Health Waters, Inc.
282 Hudson Street
Hackensack, NJ 07601
(201)489-4700

H-P Distributors
P.O. Box 233
Scottsdale, GA 30079
(404)297-0967

International Specialty Supply
820 East 20th Street
Cookeville, TN 38501
(615)526-1106

Island Natural, Inc.
559 Milford Street
Brooklyn, NY 11208
(718)272-4600

Koster
2721 East Almond Unit B
Orange, CA 92669
(714)633-5341

Kramer Food Company
P.O. Box 7033
Troy, MI 48007-7033
(313)585-8141

Maranatha Natural Foods
P.O. Box 1046
Ashland, OR 97520
(503)488-2747

Maui Style Wholesale Ntrl. Foods
250 South Waiehu Beach Road
Wakuku, HI 96793
(808)242-4797

Meadow Farm Foods
Route 3 Box 310
Fergus Falls, MN 56537
(218)739-4585

Mountain People's Warehouse
12745 Earhart Avenue
Auburn, CA 95602
(916)889-9531

Natural Foods, Inc.
3040 Hill Avenue
P.O. Box 3267
Toledo, OH 43607
(419)537-1713

Natural Foods Northwest
East Powell Boulevard
P.O. Box 804
Gresham, OR 97030
(503)658-2169

Nature's Best
P.O. Box 2248
Brea, CA 92622-2248
(714)441-2378

Neshaminy Valley Natural Foods
Gingko Industrial Park
4 Louise Drive
Ivyland, PA 18974
(215)443-5545

Northbest Natural Products
P.O. Box 31029
Seattle, WA 98103
(206)633-2283

North Coast Foods
18660 Old Coast Hwy
Fort Bragg, CA 95437
(707)964-8332

Northeast Cooperatives
P.O. Box 8188
Brattleboro, VT 05304
(802)257-5856

North Farm Cooperative
204 Regas Road
Madison, WI 53714
(608)241-2667

Nutra Source
4005 - 6th Avenue South
Seattle, WA 98108
(206)467-7190

O-Jib-Wa Vitamin Co.
2901 East Court Street
Flint, MI 48506
(313)232-5839

Orange Blossom Coop Warehouse
1601 NW 55th Place
P.O. Box 4159
Gainesville, FL 32613
(904)372-7061

Ozark Cooperative Warehouse
P.O. Box 1528
Fayetteville, AR 71702-1528
(501)521-2667

Palko Distributing Company
792 Mccool Road
Valparaiso, IN 46383
(219)759-1199

P.N.Q.
1450 Pennsylvania Avenue
Allentown, PA 18103
(215)694-0333

Quong Hop & Co.
161 Beacon Street
South San Francisco, CA 94080
(415)761-2022

Rainbow Distributing, Inc.
2718 North Paulina
Chicago, IL 60614
(312)929-7629

Ray's Food Services, Inc.
P.O. Box 919
Clackamas, OR 97015
(503)655-1177

Rosewood Products, Inc.
738 Airport Boulevard Suite 6
Ann Arbor, MI 48108
(313)665-2222

Shojin Natural Food, Inc.
P.O. Box 247
Kealakekua, HI 96759
(808)322-3651

Specialty Health Foods
1917 West Howard
Chicago, IL 60626
(312)274-4899

Stow Mills
P.O. Box 301
Chesterfield, NH
(603)256-3000

Sun Ray Products Distribution
Div. Tree of Life, Inc.
570 NE 185th Street
Miami, FL 33179
(305)653-5412

Sunshower Farm
48548 - 60th Avenue
Lawrence, MI 49064
(616)674-3103

Tochi Products
1107 Second Avenue North
P.O. Box 2215
Fargo, ND 58108
(701)232-7717

Tree of Life Midwest
P.O. Box 2629
Bloomington, IN 47402
(800)999-4200

Tree of Life, Northeast
2501 - 71st Street
North Bergen, NJ 07047
(201)662-7200

Tree of Life Northwest
7036 South 190th Street
Kent, WA 98032
(206)251-5220

Tree of Life Southeast
1750 Tree Boulevard
P.O. Box 410
St. Augustine, FL 32085
(904)824-8181

Tree of Life/Southwest Div.
105 Bluebonnet Drive
Cleburne, TX 76031
(817)641-6678

Tree of Life West
9501 El Dorado Avenue
Sylmar, CA 91352
(818)768-2330

U.T.D. Company
762 Industrial Drive
Elmhurst, IL 60126
(800)878-7990

Tucson Co-op Warehouse
350 South Toole Avenue
Tucson, AZ 85701
(602)884-9951

Vitality Distributors, Inc.
1010 NW 51st Place
Ft. Lauderdale, FL 33309
(305)944-0391

Preferred Brands

When a person begins to change what he or she eats, one of the most overwhelming jobs is grocery shopping. The familiar brands go by the wayside. But, how does one begin to shop for new brands? Our family has found the following brands to taste good, be reasonably priced, and contain quality ingredients. It is important to support companies that are committed to quality products, so that we can do our part to keep them in business.

This list is not all-inclusive, but it does contain the brands that we use on a regular basis. I am sure you will find these brands to be a good place to start. No company has paid for these recommendations. I am simply passing on our preferences after years of experimentation.

If you are unable to find these products in your stores, you may want to ask that they carry them. Some companies allow you to order directly. Many have free recipe booklets and brochures on their products.

Alta Dena has a great line of quality dairy products, from fresh milk to kefir, yoghurt, ice cream, and others. They are committed to producing milk products without bovine growth hormones. Dairy products without this hormone are much safer for you and your family. Alta Dena's quality and integrity are excellent.

> Alta Dena Certified Dairy
> P.O. Box 388
> City-Industry, CA 91747-0388
> (818)964-6401
> (800)535-1369

Annie's produces excellent dressings and barbecue sauces. Their dressings and sauces are just like homemade—fresh and tasty. Try their barbecue sauce on oven-fried potatoes. The raspberry dressing is one of our family's favorites.

> Annie's
> Foster Hill Road
> North Calais, VT 05650
> (802)456-8866

Arrowhead Mills is a wonderful manufacturer that will easily replace many all-purpose brands that you currently purchase. Virtually all their products are organic with great taste and include whole grains, flours, mixes, beans, seeds, nut and seed butters (they have excellent tahini), oils, flakes, and soup mixes.

> Arrowhead Mills, Inc.
> 110 South Lawton
> Box 2059
> Hereford, TX 79045
> (806)364-0730

Barbara's Bakery provides quality nutritional and snack foods, from chips, pretzels, and cookies to cereals, granola bars, bread sticks, and crackers. Their food is tasty and very reasonably priced.

Barbara's Bakery, Inc.
3900 Cypress Drive
Petaluma, CA 94954
(707)765-2273

Cascadian Farms provides a wealth of excellent products. Many of their products are organic, from their frozen fruits and vegetables to their jams, jellies, preserves, sorbets, pickles, and relishes. They have great "popsicles" made with organic milk and unrefined sugar. Kosher foods are also available.

Cascadian Farms
P.O. Box 568
Concrete, WA 98237
phone: (206)855-0100   fax: (206)855-0444

Celestial Seasonings produces the finest line of herbal teas. They now have a line of black teas and gourmet after-dinner teas.

Celestial Seasonings
4600 Sleepytime Drive
Boulder, CO 80020
(303)530-5300

Cold Mountain Miso (white miso) can be found in the dairy sections of most health-food stores. The lighter the color of the miso, the milder the flavor. Miso is a great replacement for traditional bouillon cubes.

Cold Mountain Miso
Miyako Oriental Foods Inc.
4287 Puente Avenue
Baldwin Park, CA 91706
phone: (818)962-9633   fax: (818)814-4569

Coleman Natural Meats are totally natural and raised without hormones or steroids. The flavor is excellent, beyond comparison to other commercially available meats. They provide beef and some other meats.

Coleman Natural Meats Inc.
5140 Race Court #4
Denver, CO 80127
phone: (303)297-9393   fax: (303)297-0426

DeBoles Pasta is a good transition pasta for families just beginning to change their diet. Pastas are made with semolina and Jerusalem artichoke flour. They also provide some corn pasta and other bakery products.

DeBoles Nutritional Foods, Inc.
2120 Jericho Turnpike
Garden City Park, NY 11040
(516)742-1818

Eden produces excellent vinegars, along with many other Asian foods, tomato products, pastas, beans, and soy milks. Many products are organic. Their brand names include Eden, Edensoy, and Herbs Pasta.

Eden Foods, Inc.
701 Tecumseh
Clinton, MI 49236
(517)456-7424

Fantastic Foods has one of the best lines of packaged foods. They produce natural convenience food (dry mixes), grains, cereals, and soups. They also have kosher foods. Their brand names include Fantastic Falafil, Nature's Burger (great vegetarian hamburger replacement), Quick Pilafs, Instant Refried Beans, Fantastic Noodles, and Meals In A Cup.

Fantastic Foods
1250 North McDowell Boulevard
Petaluma, CA 94954
(707)778-7801

Frontier provides fresh herbs in bulk and packaged forms. They also produce organic coffees. This company is committed to quality and integrity.

> Frontier Cooperatives Herbs
> 1 Frontier Road
> P.O. Box 299
> Norway, IA 52318
> (800)669-3275

FruitSource is a balanced sweetener made from brown rice and grapes that many diabetics can use. It comes in both liquid and granular forms. It can be used one for one in sugar replacement.

> FruitSource
> 1803 Mission Street Suite 404
> Santa Cruz, CA 95060
> (408)457-1136

Garden of Eatin' has a wide variety of chips. I have found that many people do better with the blue or red corn chips instead of the yellow. They also have excellent pita breads, bagels, tortillas, *chapatis*, and sprouted rolls. Certified organic ingredients are included in most products.

> Garden of Eatin'
> 5300 Santa Monica Boulevard
> Los Angeles, CA 90029
> (213)462-5406

Glenny's produces an alternative to candy with sugar. From lollipops to snack bars, their products are a great alternative. Brand names include Nookies, Noah 'N Friends Animal Cookies, and Glenny's.

> Glenny's 100% Natural Snacks
> 999 Central Avenue
> Woodmere, NY 11598
> (no phone listed)

Guiltless Gourmet has excellent fat-free snacks including baked, no-oil chips. Their fat-free bean dips and salsas are excellent and some of our favorites.

Guiltless Gourmet
3709 Promontory Point Drive, Suite 131
Austin, TX 78744
(512)443-4373

Hatch provides great Mexican foods, from salsas to chilies, refried beans (both pinto and black bean), and taco shells. Their green chili enchilada sauce (vegetarian) is excellent.

Hatch Chili Company
P.O. Box 752
Deming, NM 88031
(505)546-4298

Imagine Foods makes three delicious brands, including Rice Dream, Ken & Robert's, and Veggie Pockets. Rice Dream is a food product made from the starch portion of brown rice. It is a delicious milk that can be used for drinking, cooking, and baking. It is also available in frozen "ice-cream"–type products. Ken & Robert's is a brand of delicious frozen vegetarian entrees. Veggie Pockets are frozen vegetarian pocket sandwiches, individually frozen for quick meals.

Imagine Foods
350 Cambridge Avenue Suite 350
Palo Alto, CA 94306
phone: (415)327-1444   fax: (415)327-1459

Knudsen & Sons has great juices, carbonated beverages, syrups, and spreads. Their products are an excellent replacement for sugar-sweetened colas and carbonated beverages.

Knudsen & Sons
P.O. Box 369
Chico, CA 95927
(916)891-1517

KyoGreen products have become a daily staple in our home. From Kyolic (aged garlic) to KyoGreen, we use each product to build our immune system and help maintain overall strong body systems. KyoGreen is added to our fruit smoothies each morning. Kyolic garlic is a regular supplement throughout the year, especially during the fall and winter.

Wakunuaga of America Co., Ltd.
23501 Madero
Mission Viejo, CA 92691
(714)855-2776

Lundberg produces organic and premium brown-rice products. They also have rice blends, brown-rice cakes, flours, cereals, pilafs. Their brown-rice syrup is an excellent sugar replacement that many diabetics can use. Their brown-rice pudding mixes are excellent.

Lundberg Family Farms
P.O. Box 369
Richvale, CA 95974
(916)882-4551

Maine Coast Sea Vegetables offers a full line of sea vegetables or seaweed. Adding that strip of kombu to your soups or beans aids in digestion and intake of minerals.

Maine Coast Sea Vegetables
Shore Road
Franklin, MA 04630
(207)565-2907

Mom's Spaghetti Sauce is one of our all-time favorite sauces on our homemade pasta. It has big chunks of fresh basil and whole cloves of garlic. A truly delicious sauce.

Mom's Spaghetti Sauce
Timpone's Fresh Foods Corp.
3211 Thornton B
Austin, TX 78704
(512)442-7772

Mori Nu has the best silken tofu (a smooth tofu with the texture of sour cream, without the cholesterol). It works the best with many of my recipes. It comes in aseptic packaging for longer shelf life. Their new "lite" tofu has the least amount of fat of any tofu on the market.

Mori Nu
Morinaga Nutritional Foods, Inc.
5800 Eastern Avenue, Suite 270
Los Angeles, CA 90040
(213)728-4325

Mountain Sun is committed to organic products. They provide great organic and natural food juices under the labels of Mountain Sun and Apple Hill.

Mountain Sun
18390 Hwy 145
Dolores, CO 81323
phone: (303)882-2283   fax: (303)882-2270

Muir Glen tomato products are by far my favorite. These organically grown tomato products are packaged in enamel-lined cans, which produces a superior taste and product. Their products range from chunky sauces to paste to whole tomatoes. Throw away those tinny-tasting tomatoes and try Muir Glen.

Muir Glen
424 North 7th Street
Sacramento, CA 95814
(916)557-0900

Nayonaise produces a dairy-free mayo made from tofu. They also make tofu dressings, wonton skins, egg roll wrappers, and tofu.

Nasoya Foods Inc.
23 Jytek Drive
Leominster, MA 01453
(508)537-0713

Nest Eggs provides eggs from uncaged hens that are fed a drug-free diet. Quality eggs are just as important as organic grains, produce, and meats.

Nest Eggs Inc.
P.O. Box 14599
Chicago, IL 60614
(no phone listed)

Pamela's Products produces our favorite cookies. Many of their cookies are wheat-free (wheat is the most common American food allergy) and low in fat. All cookies are sugar-free.

Pamela's Products
156 Utah Avenue
South San Francisco, CA 94080
(415)952-4546

Parsley Patch provides an excellent line of salt-free seasonings. Their Mexican Blend is a staple for my Mexican dishes.

Parsley Patch
McCormick & Co., Inc.
Hunt Valley, MD 21031-1100
(410)771-7301

Roaster Fresh makes excellent nut butters. They are produced by Kettel Foods, which also makes chips, popcorn, and other nuts and seeds.

Roaster Fresh/Kettle Foods
P.O. Box 664
Salem, OR 97308
(503)364-0399

San-J has great sauces for stir-fries and marinades. Their tamari has an excellent flavor and will quickly replace your sodium-laden soy sauces. Their Thai peanut sauce is great for stir-fries and in salads.

San-J International, Inc.
2880 Sprouse Dr.
Richmond, VA 23231
(804)226-8333

Shady Maple Farms produces pure maple syrup that is formaldehyde-free. Pure maple syrup is far superior to the cheaper syrup mixes.

Shady Maple Farms
P.O. Box 1415
Novato, CA 94948
(no phone listed)

Sharon's Finest produces Tofu-rella, a line of soy cheese for those with dairy sensitivities. The full line of Rella cheeses works as great alternatives to dairy-based cheese.

Sharon's Finest
P.O. Box 5020
Santa Rosa, CA 95402
(707)576-7050

Shelton products, poultry, are raised without antibiotics and are free-range grown. They are also raised without hormones, or growth stimulants, which are common in most other commercially raised chickens and turkeys. ("All Natural" on a poultry label is defined by the Department of Agriculture as "minimally processed with no artificial ingredients." This claim on a whole bird only means that the bird has not been artificially basted, which is basically meaningless. Shelton provides fresh poultry and other poultry-related products. Their chicken broth is excellent.

> Shelton Poultry
> 204 Loranne
> Pomona, CA 91767
> (909)623-4361

Sno-Pac provides a line of reasonably priced, organic frozen vegetables. Out with the old brands, loaded with chemicals, and in with Sno-Pac.

> Sno-Pac Foods Inc.
> 379 S. Pine Street
> Caledonia, MN 55921
> (507)724-5281

Spectrum Naturals is my first choice for oils and has been for years. All of their oils are expeller pressed without solvents. Both refined and unrefined oils are available. Their products range from oils, supplemental oils (for example, flaxseed oil, which is a great supplemental oil to add to fruit smoothie drinks or on salads), cheese, mayonnaise, vinegars, dressings, and sauces. Their brand names include Spectrum Naturals (oils), Veg-Omega, Sonnet Farms (cheese), Ayla's Organic (dressings), and Blue Banner.

> Spectrum Naturals, Inc.
> 133 Copeland Street
> Petaluma, CA 94952
> phone: (707)778-8900   fax: (707)765-1026

Sunspire Chips is your answer to sugar-laden chocolate. Sunspire products contain no refined sugar and have a great taste. They can be purchased in carob, chocolate, mint, and peanut.

Sunspire
2114 Adams Avenue
San Leandro, CA 94577
(510)569-9731

VitaSpelt produces some of the best whole-grain pastas. They use whole-grain spelt, which many wheat-sensitive people can tolerate. Be sure to not overcook whole-grain pasta, as that will make it mushy. I have prepared many recipes for VitaSpelt products (with the brand name of Lifestyle for Health).

VitaSpelt
Purity Foods Inc.
2871 West Jolly Road
Okemos, MI 48864
(517)351-9231

Westbrae and Little Bear are two excellent brands. The company is committed to organic and low-fat products. Little Bear, under the brand name Bearitos, has excellent chips, taco shells, tostada shells, popcorn, salsa, refried beans, pretzels. They also produce a licorice without refined sugar and additives.

Little Bear/Westbrae
1065 East Walnut Street
Carson, CA 90746
(310)886-8200

Seasonal Food Chart

Food purchased during its peak season will be less expensive and much tastier. The following tables are a guideline as to which fruits and vegetables are in season each month. Use these tables to guide your menu planning.

January	February	March
Avocados	Avocados	Artichokes
Bananas	Bananas	Asparagus
Cabbage	Broccoli	Avocados
Cauliflower	Cabbage	Bananas
Mushrooms	Cauliflower	Broccoli
Pears	Kumquats	Grapefruit
Potatoes	Mangoes	Kumquats
Turnips	Mushrooms	Lettuce
Winter squash	Pears	Mushrooms
	Tangerines	Radishes
	Winter squash	Spinach

April	May	June	
Asparagus	Asparagus	Apricots	Limes
Bananas	Bananas	Avocados	Mangoes
Cabbage	Celery	Bananas	Nectarines
Escarole	Papaya	Cantaloupe	Onions
Onions	Peas	Cherries	Peaches
Pineapple	Pineapple	Corn	Peas
Radishes	Potatoes	Cucumbers	Peppers
Rhubarb	Strawberries	Figs	Pineapple
Spinach	Tomatoes	Green Beans	Plums
Strawberries	Watercress		

July	August	September
Apricots	Apples	Apples
Bananas	Bananas	Bananas
Blueberries	Beets	Broccoli
Cabbage	Berries	Carrots
Cantaloupe	Cabbage	Cauliflower
Cherries	Carrots	Corn
Corn	Corn	Cucumbers
Cucumbers	Cucumbers	Dill
Dill	Dill	Figs
Eggplant	Eggplant	Grapes
Figs	Figs	Greens
Green beans	Melons	Melons
Nectarines	Nectarines	Okra
Okra	Peaches	Onions
Peaches	Pears	Pears
Peppers	Peppers	Potatoes
Prunes	Plums	Summer squash
Watermelon	Potatoes	Tomatoes
	Summer squash	Yams
	Tomatoes	

October	November	December
Apples	Apples	Apples
Bananas	Bananas	Avocados
Broccoli	Broccoli	Bananas
Grapes	Cabbage	Grapefruit
Peppers	Cauliflower	Lemons
Persimmons	Cranberries	Limes
Pumpkin	Dates	Mushrooms
Yams	Eggplant	Oranges
	Mushrooms	Pears
	Pumpkin	Pineapple
	Sweet potatoes	Tangerines

Equivalents and Substitutions

Fruit Equivalents

Apples: 3 medium = 1 lb. = 3 c. sliced

Bananas: 3 medium = 1 lb. = 2 c. sliced = 1 c. mashed

Dates: 1 lb. = 3 c. chopped

Lemon: 1 medium = 2 to 3 tb. juice, 2 tsp. lemon zest

Lime: 1 medium = 1½ to 2 tb. juice, 1 tsp. lime zest

Orange: 1 medium = ½ c. juice, 2 tb. orange zest

Peach: 1 medium = ½ c. sliced

Pear: 1 medium = ½ c. sliced

Raisins: 1 lb. = 3 c.

Strawberries: 1 qt. = 4 c. sliced

Grain Equivalents

Cornmeal: 1 lb. = 3 c.

Flaked cereal: 3 c. dry = 1 c. crushed

Oats: 1 c. = 1¾ c. cooked

Rice: 1 c. = 3 to 4 c. cooked

Nut Equivalents
Almonds: 1 lb. unshelled = 1¾ c. nutmeat
1 lb. shelled = 3½ c. nutmeat

Peanuts:　1 lb. unshelled = 1¾ c. nutmeat
1 lb. shelled = 3½ c. nutmeat

Pecans:　1 lb. unshelled = 1¾ c. nutmeat
1 lb. shelled = 3½ c. nutmeat

Walnuts:　1 lb. unshelled = 1¾ c. nutmeat
1 lb. shelled = 3½ c. nutmeat

Vegetable Equivalents
Cabbage: 1 lb. = 3 c. shredded

Corn: 2 medium ears = 1 c. kernels

Mushrooms: 8 oz. = 3 c. raw = 1 c. sliced, cooked

Onion: 1 medium = ½ c. chopped

Pepper, green: 1 large = 1 c. diced

Potato (sweet): 3 medium = 3 c. sliced

Potato (white): 3 medium = 2 c. cubed, cooked = 1¾ c. mashed

Other Equivalents
Carob chips: 12 oz. = 2 c.

Carob powder: 1 lb. = 4 c.

Coconut: 1 lb. = 5 c. flaked or shredded

Milk cheese, raw: 1 lb. = 4 c. shredded

Pasta: 4 oz. = 1 c. = 2¼ c. cooked

General Equivalents

3 tsp. = 1 tb.   16 fluid oz. = 2 c. = 1 pt.
2 tb. (liquid) = 1 oz.   ⅛ c. = 2 tb.
4 tb. = ¼ c.   ⅓ c. = 5 tb. + 1 tsp.
5⅓ tb. = ⅓ c.   ⅔ c. = 10 tb. + 2 tsp.
8 tb. = ½ c.   4 c. = 1 qt.
16 tb. = 1 c.   4 qts. = 1 gal.
8 fluid oz. = 1 c.

Substitutes

Baking powder: use two parts cream of tartar, one part baking soda, and two parts arrowroot

Bread crumbs: toasted oats, sesame seeds, cooked brown rice, or other cracked grains

Butter: in baking use canola oil, safflower oil, sunflower oil, or applesauce (up to ½ c. per recipe)
    1 tb. = 1 tsp. light miso plus 2 tsp. olive oil for mashed
    potatoes

Buttermilk: 1 c. = 1 c. minus 1 tb. of soy milk, rice milk, or almond milk, plus 1 tb. lemon juice

Cheese: use equal amounts of soy or almond cheeses

Cheese, cottage cheese
    1 lb. firm tofu, mashed
    1 tb. olive oil
    1 tb. rice or apple-cider vinegar
    2 tb. lemon juice
    ¼ to ½ tsp. onion powder, to taste
    ¼ to ½ tsp. salt or tamari, to taste
Mix half of tofu and remaining ingredients in blender. Mix in remaining mashed tofu.

Cheese, cream cheese = "yo" cheese. Strain yoghurt in yoghurt strainer, or coffee filter placed in strainer, for twenty-four hours (set in refrigerator while draining).

Cheese, ricotta
    1 lb. firm tofu, mashed
    ¼ c. olive oil
    ½ tsp. nutmeg
    ½ tsp. salt or tamari
Mix half of tofu and remaining ingredients in blender. Mix in remaining tofu.

Chocolate: 1 square or 1 oz. = 3 tb. carob plus 1 tb. oil and 1 tb. water

Cocoa: 1 c. = 1 c. carob powder

Cornstarch: 1 tb. = 1 tb. arrowroot powder

Cream, heavy = 1 tb. tahini dissolved in ¼ c. water
(this will not whip)

Cream, sour = "yo" cheese or equal amount of soft tofu

Currants = raisins

Eggs: one egg = 1 tb. soy flour
    1 tb. water plus 1 tb. powdered soy lecithin
    commercial egg replacer
    half of a ripe banana
    4 oz. firm tofu
    ¼ c. applesauce
    ¼ c. "yo" cheese

Flour, white (as sauce thickener): 1 tb. = ½ tb. arrowroot powder

Flour, white (in baking)
    1 c. = 1 c. corn flour

1 c. = ¾ c. coarse cornmeal
1 c. = ⅞ c. rice flour
1 c. = 1 c. spelt flour
1 c. = 1 c. kamut flour
1 c. = ½ c. barley flour + ¼ c. rice flour + ½ tb. arrowroot
powder

Garlic: 1 clove = 1 tsp. minced garlic
  ½ tsp. garlic powder

Milk: 1 c. = 1 c. almond milk, soy milk, rice milk
  1 c. water plus 1 tb. tahini, mixed

Milk, sour: 1 c. = 1 tb. lemon juice or vinegar plus 1 c. less 1 tb.
milk. Let set 5 minutes.

Pepper: 1 tsp. black pepper = ¼ tsp. cayenne

Sugar, brown
  1 c. = ½ c. date sugar and ½ c. honey
  1 c. = ½ to ¾ c. honey
  1 c. = ¾ c. maple syrup
(use ½ c. less liquid per cup sweetener and reduce oven temperature by 25 degrees)

Sugar, white
  1 c. = 1 c. FruitSource
  1 c. = ¾ c. to 1 c. Sucanat
  1 c. = ¾ c. maple syrup (use 2 tb. less liquid in recipe)
  1 c. = ¾ c. honey (use 2 tb. less liquid per cup of honey used
and lower oven temperature by 25 degrees)
  1 c. = 1 c. rice syrup
  1 c. = 1 c. molasses plus ½ tsp. baking soda (use ¼ c. less
liquids per 1 c. of molasses)

Worcestershire sauce: 3 tb. = ¼ c. tamari

Yoghurt = equal amount of tofu

Newsletters and Magazines

HealthQuarters Newsletter (no charge)
6873 Prince Drive
Colorado Springs, CO 80918
(719)593-8694

Herb Companion ($21/year)
Interweave Press, Inc.
201 East Fourth Street
Loveland, CO 80537

Lifestyle for Health Newsletter ($20/year)
P.O. Box 3871
Littleton, CO 80161-3871
    Send a SASE (legal size) for one complimentary issue. Edited by Cheryl Townsley.

Organic Advocate
Albert's Organics
Publications Department
4605 South Alameda Street
Los Angeles, CA 90058

Total Health ($13/year)
Trio Publications
6001 Topanaga Canyon Boulevard #300
Woodland Hills, CA 91367

Vegetarian Journal ($20/year)
Vegetarian Resource Group
P.O. Box 1463
Baltimore, MD 21203

Vegetarian Times ($16/eight months)
P.O. Box 570
Oak Park, IL 60303
(800)892-0753

For a national list of nutritional professionals, contact:

HealthQuarters Nutritional Resource List
6873 Prince Drive
Colorado Springs, CO 80918
(Reference guide is available for $25/tax-deductible.)

APPENDIX G

Books

Bailey, Covert. *Fit or Fat?* Boston, MA: Houghton Mifflin, 1989.

Baker, Elizabeth and Elton. *Bandwagon to Health.* Saguache, CO: Drelwood Publications, 1982.

Ballentine, Rudolph. *Diet and Nutrition.* Honesdale, PA: Himalayan Publishers, n.d.

Bieler, Henry G., and Maxine Block. *Food Is Your Best Medicine.* New York: Ballantine Books, 1987.

Calborn, Cherie, and Maureen Keane. *Juicing for Life.* Garden City Park, NY: Avery Publishing, 1992.

Cousins, Norman. *Anatomy of an Illness as Perceived by the Patient.* New York: Bantam Books, 1983.

Crook, William G. *The Yeast Connection.* Jackson, TN: Professional Books, 1988.

Diamond, Harvey and Marilyn. *Fit for Life.* New York: Warner Books, 1985.

Diamond, Harvey and Marilyn. *Fit for Life II*. New York: Warner Books, 1988.

Eckhardt, Linda W. *Satisfaction Guaranteed: Simply Sumptuous Mail Order Foods with Recipes and Menus for Fast and Fabulous Meals*. New York: Jeremy P. Tarcher, 1986.

Erasmus, Udo. *Fats and Oils*. Burnaby, BC: Alive Books, 1986.

Frähm, Anne E. and David J. *A Cancer Battle Plan*. Colorado Springs, CO: Piñon Press, 1992.

Frähm, Anne E., and David J. *Healthy Habits*. Colorado Springs, CO: Piñon Press, 1993.

Jensen, Bernard. *Foods That Heal*. Garden City Park, NY: Avery Publishing Group, 1988.

Jensen, Bernard. *Tissue Cleaning Through Bowel Management*. Escondido, CA: Bernard Jensen, 1981.

Kadans, Joseph. *Encyclopedia of Fruits, Vegetables, Nuts, and Seeds for Healthful Living*. Englewood Cliffs, NJ: Reward Books, 1975.

Kloss, Jethro. *Back to Eden*. Loma Linda, CA: Back to Eden Books, 1985.

Null, Gary. *Gary Null's Complete Guide to Healing Your Body Naturally*. New York: McGraw-Hill, 1988.

Quillin, Patrick. *Healing Nutrients*. New York: Random House, 1989.

Reuben, David. *Everything You Always Wanted to Know About Nutrition*. New York: Avon, 1979.

Robbins, John. *Diet for a New America*. Walpole, NH: Stillpoint Publishing, 1987.

Salaman, Maureen. *Nutrition: The Cancer Answer*. Statford, CA: Statford Publishing, 1984.

Santillo, Humbart. *Natural Healing with Herbs*. Prescott, AZ: Hohm Press, 1990.

Tenney, Louise. *Today's Herbal Health*. Provo, UT: Woodland Books, 1992.

Walker, N. W., D.Sc. *Fresh Vegetable and Fruit Juices*. Prescott, AZ: Norwalk Press, 1970.

Wigmore, Ann. *The Wheatgrass Book*. Wayne, NJ: Avery Publishing, 1985.

Cookbooks

Barkie, Karen E. *Sweet and Sugarfree*. New York: St. Martin's Press, 1982.

Bingham, Rita. *Country Beans*. Edmond, OK: Natural Meals in Minutes, 1989.

Blackman, Jackson F. *Working Chef's Cookbook for Natural Whole Foods*. Morrisville, VT: Central VT Publishers, 1989.

Diamond, Marilyn. *The American Vegetarian Cookbook from the Fit for Life Kitchen*. New York: Warner Books, 1990.

DuBelle, Lee. *Proper Food Combining Cookbook*. Phoenix, AZ: Walsh & Associates, 1984.

Dumke, Nicolette M. *Allergy Cooking with Ease*. Lancaster, PA: Starburst Publishers, 1992.

Elliot, Rose. *Complete Vegetarian Cuisine*. New York: Pantheon, 1988.

Gerras, Charles. *Rodale's Basic Natural Foods Cookbook*. Emmaus, PA: Rodale Press, 1984.

Katzen, Mollie. *Mososewood Cookbook*. Berkeley, CA: Ten Speed Press, 1987.

Killeen, Jacquieline. *The Whole World Cookbook*. New York: Charles Scribner's Sons, 1979.

McCarty, Meredith. *Fresh from a Vegetarian Kitchen*. Eureka, CA: Turning Point Publications, 1990.

Robertson, Laurel. *The New Laurel's Kitchen*. Berkeley, CA: Ten Speed Press, 1986.

Romano, Rita. *Dining in the Raw*. Prato, Italy: Prato Publishing, 1992.

Townsley, Cheryl. *Kid's Favorites*. Denver, CO: self-published, 1992.

Townsley, Cheryl. *Lifestyle for Health*. Denver, CO: self-published, 1991.

Townsley, Cheryl. *Meals in 30 Minutes*. Denver, CO: self-published, 1992.

Wood, Rebecca. *The Whole Foods Encyclopedia: A Shopper's Guide*. New York: Prentice-Hall, 1988.

Glossary

GENERAL GLOSSARY

ADZUKI BEAN: a sprouting bean, similar to a MUNG BEAN, but usually less expensive. It is chewy and if cooked, requires more time. In many Asian countries it is believed to be healing for the kidneys.

AGAR-AGAR FLAKES: a dried extract from sea plants. High in minerals, it acts as a natural laxative. It is used to congeal or thicken. Use two teaspoons dissolved in half a cup of hot, not boiling, water for molded salad, and two to three times that amount for "finger" treats.

AMAZAKE: a milk made from sweet brown rice. Excellent for children and infants. High in CALCIUM. Can be diluted to substitute for milk in cooking. Flavored varieties are excellent to drink.

ARROWROOT POWDER: a starch from the root of a tropical plant used to thicken sauces, soups. Good substitute for corn-starch.

BOK CHOY: Chinese green leafy vegetable with thick, juicy stalks. Delicious in stir-fry.

BRAGGS AMINO ACIDS: a light alternative to soy sauce. It is made with soybeans and water.

BUCKWHEAT: a fruit, not a grain, that has many uses. White buckwheat GROATS can be ground into flour for a milder buckwheat flour. Makes wonderful sprouts. It is full of vitamins, minerals, complete protein, and enzymes. Roasted buckwheat, called KASHA, is also available in unroasted form.

BULGUR: a food prepared from whole wheat that is cracked, steamed, and dried.

BURDOCK: edible parts are the young leaves, roots, and stems. The roots are blood and kidney purifiers. It is higher in minerals than BEETS, CARROTS, POTATOES, or turnips.

CANOLA OIL: an oil low in saturated fat and easily digested. It is one of the mildest flavored oils and, therefore, preferred in baked products.

CAROB: sweet and similar to chocolate without the side effects, it is a natural substitute for chocolate or cocoa. It does not produce the negative effects of caffeine, theo-bromine, and calcium oxylate. Roasted CAROB is not as nutritious as raw carob.

CHICKPEAS: also called garbanzo beans, these nutty-flavored beans are good cooked or sprouted.

COUSCOUS: a traditional grain made from semi-refined wheat. It can be used for main-course dishes or desserts.

DAIKON: a long, large Japanese white radish. It is believed to help dissolve animal-fat deposits found in the body.

DULSE: (dried) purple sea vegetable or sea weed. Twelve times more nutritious than the average vegetable. Wash, soak a few minutes, and add to salads. Wash, re-dry, and grind into a coarse powder and use for seasoning. It is high in IRON, VITAMIN A, and PHOSPHORUS.

FLAXSEED: has the highest content of VITAMIN E of any known seed. It excels in complete bulk fiber, is easy to digest, is high in complete protein, and rich in minerals and oil. It can be used as a thickener in cookies, dressing, etc. It has a satisfying, nutlike flavor.

GINGER: a pungent root used in many ways. It is believed to increase circulation and the breakdown of fats in the body.

GOMASIO: a delicious condiment using roasted sesame seeds and sea salt. One part salt and fourteen parts sesame seeds, ground, make gomasio. It can be used in place of salt. It adds salt, protein, CALCIUM, and flavor.

GRITS: coarsely ground hulled grain.

GROATS: a coarser grind of hulled grain than GRITS.

HUMMUS: a Middle Eastern food, usually made from puréed CHICKPEAS, TAHINI garlic, and lemon juice.

JERUSALEM ARTICHOKES: a root vegetable with a crunchy taste. It can be used in place of water chestnuts. It is believed to be very cleansing and balancing.

JICAMA: a roundish root vegetable. The pulp is sweet, juicy, and crunchy. It can be used in salads or stir-fries.

KASHA: a Russian dish of cooked BUCKWHEAT. Another name for hulled buckwheat grains before being cooked.

KELP: rich in IODINE and other minerals. Kelp can be used instead of salt.

KOMBU: a broad, thick seaweed. It is rich in minerals and often used in cooking soup stocks or beans.

KUZU (KUDZU): extracted from the root of the kuzu vine. It is a white, lumpy starch with a high IRON content, plus large amounts of CALCIUM, PHOSPHORUS, and sodium. Used to gel liquids. One tablespoon will thicken a cup to gravy consistency. Two and a half tablespoons will thicken a cup to a gelatinlike mass when cooled. Kuzu has no taste of its own.

LECITHIN: a substance that is composed of two B vitamins and oil that occurs naturally in soybeans. It can be used to coat baking pans to prevent sticking, or in baking and salad dressings for increased VITAMIN B.

MILLET: a small yellow grain that is alkaline instead of acidic in the body. One of the most balancing of the grains.

MISO: a fermented paste from grains and/or beans. It is fermented in wooden barrels for twelve to thirty-six months. It is generally used as a soup base or flavoring agent. The darker the color, the stronger the flavor. It is protein-rich and believed to be beneficial to the circulatory as well as the digestive organs.

MOLASSES: a highly mineral-rich sweetener.

MUNG BEAN THREADS: found in Asian markets or health-food stores. A type of pasta is made from MUNG BEANS—a suitable substitute for pasta made from grains.

PSYLLIUM SEED HUSKS: used as a thickening agent, they are an excellent source of dietary fiber. Finely ground husks can be used as a food thickener.

RICE MILK: a milk made from brown rice.

RICE PAPER: a thin paperlike dough made from rice. Similar to phyllo or wonton wrappers.

RICE STICK NOODLES: pasta made from rice. Can be boiled or fried. Found in Asian markets or health-food stores.

RICE SYRUP: a sweet syrup made from brown rice. It can be used as a sweetener in cooking. Jars usually have a chart indicating the level of sweetness.

SEITEN: a wheat-gluten food that is often used to replace meat. It is high in protein and can absorb the flavor of the liquids that it cooks in.

SOBA NOODLES: thin BUCKWHEAT noodles found in many Japanese dishes. Found in Asian markets or health-food stores.

SOY MILK: a drink made from soybeans.

STEVIA: an herb from South America used as a replacement for sweeteners. It comes in liquid, powder, or a dry leaf form. It is highly concentrated and takes only about one-half to one *teaspoon* of the powder to replace one cup of sugar.

TAHINI: a butter made from either toasted or raw sesame seeds, used as a condiment or spread. Can also be used as a dairy substitute. Very high in CALCIUM.

TAMARI: a byproduct of MISO. Made from fermented soy, kozi, and unrefined sea salt. True tamari is wheat-free.

TEMPEH: a traditional, fermented food of Indonesia made from cooked soybeans inoculated with a mold starter. Used as a meat substitute. Chewier than TOFU.

TEMPURA: a Japanese dish consisting of vegetables or seafood dipped in batter and fried.

TOFU: a firm, custardlike cheese made from soybeans, water, and a solidifier.

UMEBOSHI VINEGAR: a vinegar made from the umeboshi plum. These salty-sour plums have been pickled in salt for twelve to twenty-four months. They add a great taste and aid in digestion.

WHEY: the liquid residue resulting from the coagulation of milk. It contains mostly water and some milk sugar, minerals, protein, and butterfat.

HERBS

ALLSPICE: A pea-sized fruit that grows in Mexico, Jamaica, and Central and South America. Its delicate flavor resembles a blend of cloves, cinnamon, and nutmeg.

Uses: whole—meats, boiled fish, gravies; ground—puddings, preserves, baking

ANISE: An aromatic seed from Spain and Mexico. Often used in dishes in conjunction with or to replace cinnamon.

Uses: apple dishes, chutneys, cookies, SWEET POTATOES, spice cake, SQUASH

BASIL: The dried leaves and stems of an herb grown in the United States. Has an aromatic leafy flavor.

Uses: flavoring TOMATO dishes, veggies, lamb dishes, and poultry

BAY LEAVES: The dried leaves of an evergreen grown in the eastern Mediterranean countries. Has a sweet, herbal, floral spice taste.

Uses: pickling, stews, sauces, soups

CARAWAY: The seed of a plant grown in the Netherlands. Its flavor combines the tastes of ANISE and DILL.

Uses: baking breads, often added to sauerkraut, noodles, French-fried POTATOES

CARDAMON: An aromatic pod from India, Sri Lanka, and Guatemala. It can be purchased ground or in pod form.

Uses: CURRY mixtures, fruit punches, puddings, baked goods, SWEET POTATOES

CILANTRO: A leafy herb from Spain, Italy, or Mexico. Usually used fresh; also available dry.

Uses: Chinese dishes, Italian salads and casseroles, Spanish and Latin American meat and bean dishes

CUMIN: An aromatic seed with an earthy taste. It can be purchased in seed or ground form.

Uses: Mexican dishes, soups, spicy sauces, with chili powder or CURRY POWDER

CURRY POWDER: A ground blend of GINGER, turmeric, and as many as sixteen to twenty spices.

Uses: Indian curry recipes, stir-fry

DILL: The small, dark seed of the dill plant grown in India; has a clean aromatic taste.

Uses: sauerkraut, potato salad, veggies, and soups

FENNEL: A watermelon-shaped seed with a licorice flavor.

Uses: Italian sauces, Italian breads, meat dishes

MACE: The dried covering around the nutmeg seed. Its flavor is similar to nutmeg, but with a fragrant, delicate difference.

Uses: baked goods, CAROB desserts

MARJORAM: An herb of the mint family, grown in France and Chile. It has a minty-sweet flavor.

Uses: beverages, jellies, soups, stews, sauces. Excellent sprinkled on lamb while roasting

OREGANO: A plant of the mint family and a species of MARJORAM. The dried leaves are used to make an herb seasoning.

Uses: TOMATO dishes, pizza, chili, and Italian specialties

PAPRIKA: A mild, sweet red pepper grown in Spain, Central Europe, and the United States. It is slightly aromatic and prized for its brilliant red color.

Uses: garnish for pale foods, Hungarian goulash, salad dressings

POPPY: The seed of a flower grown in Holland. It has a rich

fragrance and crunchy, nutlike flavor.

Uses: excellent as a topping for bread, cookies, or noodles

ROSEMARY: An herb (like a curved pine needle) grown in France, Spain, and Portugal; has a sweet, fresh taste.

Uses: lamb dishes, soups, stews

SAGE: The leaf of a shrub grown in Greece and the Balkans. Its flavor is savory and minty.

Uses: poultry stuffing, meat loaf, stews, and salads

THYME: The leaves and stems of a shrub grown in France and Spain. It has a strong, distinctive flavor.

Uses: poultry seasoning, croquettes, fish dishes, and TOMATOES

TURMERIC: A root of the GINGER family, grown in India, Haiti, Jamaica, and Peru. Has a mild, ginger-pepper flavor.

Uses: flavoring and coloring in mustard dishes, dressings, sauces, and salads

VITAMINS AND MINERALS

Vitamins

VITAMIN A

Functions: A is essential for maintaining membrane tissue and resisting infection in sinuses, lungs, air passages, gastrointestinal tract, vagina, and eyes. Prevents night blindness and oversensitivity to light. Promotes growth, vitality, appetite, and digestion. Helps prevent aging and senility. Helps counteract damaging effect of air pollution.

Sources: dark green leafy vegetables, orange and yellow fruits and vegetables, whole grains, sprouts, and seaweed.

Enemies: air pollutants, alcohol, coffee, cortisone, excess IRON, mineral oil, lack of sun.

VITAMIN B COMPLEX

Functions: B promotes digestion, growth, and appetite. Maintains health of nerves and brain. Necessary during nursing. Helps prevent degenerative diseases such as arthritis. Aids in protein metabolism, helps prevent tooth decay, edema, epileptic seizures.

Sources: wild rice, bran, sprouts, almonds, legumes, dark green leafy vegetables, raw fruit.

Enemies: alcohol, caffeine, coffee, sugar, tobacco, oral contraceptives, excess starches, sleeping pills, estrogen, stress, sulfa drugs.

VITAMIN C

Functions: C is essential for healthy collagen, the "glue" that holds cells together. Necessary for vital functions of all organs and glands. Protects against stress (physical and mental), toxic chemicals, and some poisons. Acts as a natural antibiotic and promotes healing. Aids in maintaining healthy sex organs and adrenal glands. Assists in healthy tooth formation.

Sources: all raw fruits and vegetables, especially red bell PEPPERS, TOMATOES, citrus fruit, green leafy vegetables, and sprouts.

Enemies: alcohol, antibiotics, aspirin, barbiturates, cooking heat, cortisone, high fevers, pain killers, stress, tobacco.

VITAMIN D

Functions: D is essential for utilization of CALCIUM and other metals by the digestive tract. Necessary for proper function of thyroid and other glands. Assures proper formation of bones and teeth in children.

Sources: exposure of uncovered skin to the sun, fish-liver oils, raw milk, egg yolks, sprouted seeds, MUSHROOMS.

Enemies: barbiturates, cortisone, mineral oil, sleeping pills, smog.

VITAMIN E

Functions: E provides oxygen to tissues and cells. Improves circulation. Prevents and reduces scar tissue. Retards aging, lessens menopausal disorders. Essential for the health of reproductive organs. Serves as an anticoagulant.

Sources: raw and sprouted seeds and grains, legumes, eggs, dark green leafy vegetables, and nuts.

Enemies: CHLORINE, heat, mineral oil, rancid fat and oils, oral contraceptives.

VITAMIN K

Functions: K is vital for blood clotting and liver function. Also aids in vitality and longevity.

Sources: seeds, sprouts, raw milk, alfalfa, KELP.

Minerals

CALCIUM

Functions: Calcium is vital for all muscle and body activity. Needed for building and maintaining bones, and for normal growth, heart action, and blood clotting. Essential for normal pregnancy and lactation. Must be present for MAGNESIUM to be utilized.

Sources: sesame seeds (more than milk), TAHINI, raw milk, dark green leafy vegetables, KELP, and sea vegetables.

Enemies: aspirin, chocolate, mineral oil, oxalic acid, stress.

CHLORINE

Functions: Chlorine aids the liver in detoxifying the body. Necessary for the production of hydrochloric acid, which is used in the stomach for digestion of proteins.

Sources: DULSE, sea vegetables, dark green leafy vegetables, AVOCADOS, oats, ASPARAGUS, TOMATOES, sea fish.

Enemies: excess rancid fats and oil.

CHROMIUM
Functions: Chromium is necessary for utilization of sweeteners. Involved with activity of hormones and enzymes. Aids in metabolism of cholesterol. Identified as glucose tolerance factor. Helps regulate serum cholesterol.

Sources: whole-grain cereal, grain sprouts, MUSHROOMS, liver.

Enemies: refined carbohydrates, sugar.

COPPER
Functions: Copper is essential for the absorption of IRON. Helps in development of bones, nerves, connective tissues, and brain. Aids protein metabolism.

Sources: legumes, leafy green vegetables, whole grains, grain sprouts, almonds, raisins, PRUNES.

Enemies: coffee, stress.

IODINE
Functions: Iodine is essential for the health and function of the thyroid gland, which regulates much of the body's activity (mental and physical). Regulates energy, body weight, and metabolism.

Sources: DULSE, KELP, green leafy vegetables, pineapple, citrus fruit, watercress, seafood.

Enemies: cooking heat, soaking in water.

IRON
Functions: Iron is necessary for formation of red blood cells, which transport oxygen to all body cells. Quality hemoglobin provides resistance to disease and stress.

Sources: blackstrap MOLASSES, raisins, PRUNES, nuts, seeds, whole grains, sea plants, sprouts, legumes.

Enemies: coffee, some food additives.

MAGNESIUM
Functions: Magnesium is essential for enzyme activity. Aids in body's use of VITAMIN B and E, fats, and other minerals, especially CALCIUM. Helps provide strong bones and muscle tone. Contributes to a healthy heart. Balances acid-alkaline condition of the body. Helps prevent buildup of cholesterol.

Sources: sesame, sunflower, pumpkin seeds; almonds; whole grains; green leafy vegetables; sprouts; APPLES; peaches; and LEMONS.

Enemies: alcohol, diuretics, food processing, refined flour, sugar, excess protein.

MANGANESE
Functions: Manganese aids in the digestion of fats. It promotes the production of sex hormones. It also strengthens tissue and bones and is used by the kidneys, liver, lymph system, pancreas, spleen, heart, and brain.

Sources: citrus fruits, APRICOTS, outer coating (not the shell) of nuts, BEETS, and CARROTS.

Enemies: excess CALCIUM and PHOSPHORUS.

PHOSPHORUS
Functions: Phosphorus promotes healthy growth of bones and teeth. It works in conjunction with CALCIUM to help metabolize fats and carbohydrates. It aids in the growth and repair of cells and nerves. Builds blood, brain, and hair.

Sources: bran, nuts, seeds, beans.

Enemies: sugar, excess aluminum, IRON, and MAGNESIUM.

POTASSIUM
Functions: Potassium aids in the pH balance in the blood and tissues. It assists in the kidney's work of detoxifying the blood. Stimulates endocrine hormone production and helps regulate the heartbeat.

Sources: seaweeds, nuts, dried fruits, legumes, bran.

Enemies: alcohol, caffeine, coffee, cortisone, many laxatives and diuretics, stress, excess salt.

SELENIUM
Functions: Selenium creates an antioxidant effect similar to VITAMIN E. Protects against mercury poisoning and preserves tissue elasticity.

Sources: bran, BROCCOLI, KELP, GARLIC, wheat germ.

Enemies: excess fats, stress.

SULFUR
Functions: Sulfur aids in digestion and counteracts acidosis. It assists in maintaining healthy hair, blood, nails, and skin. It also helps purify the blood.

Sources: RASPBERRIES, nuts, alfalfa, CABBAGES, GARLIC, dark green leafy vegetables.

Enemies: none.

ZINC
Functions: Zinc assists in healing wounds and burns. Contributes to protein and carbohydrate metabolism as well as healthy reproductive organs. It effects the transfer of carbon dioxide from the tissues to lungs.

Sources: wheat germ and bran, seeds, nuts, soy products.

Enemies: alcohol, food processing, oral contraceptives, stress, excess CALCIUM.

FRUITS AND VEGETABLES

APPLES: Apples are an alkaline and eliminative food. They contain 50 percent more VITAMIN A than ORANGES. They contain vitamin G (the "appetite vitamin"), which promotes digestion and growth. Apples are blood purifiers and therefore beneficial for low blood pressure and hardening of the arteries.

APRICOTS: Apricots are natural laxatives and rate high in alkalinity. They also contain cobalt, which is necessary to treat anemic conditions.

ARTICHOKES: Artichokes have a great deal of roughage. They are perfect to eat on a reduction diet. They contain VITAMIN A and C, CALCIUM, and IRON.

ASPARAGUS: Asparagus acts as a stimulant to the kidneys, if not taken to excess. It contains chlorophyll and is therefore an effective blood purifier. The green tips are high in VITAMIN A. Asparagus is high in water content and is considered a beneficial vegetable in an elimination diet.

AVOCADOS: Avocados contain large amounts of fruit oil, a rare element that is high in food energy and has few carbohydrates. They are high in IRON and COPPER, which aid in red blood regeneration and the prevention of anemia. They also contain sodium and POTASSIUM, which give the fruit a high alkaline reaction.

BANANAS: Bananas are easily assimilated and contain many vitamins, minerals, and a great deal of fiber. Bananas feed the natural acidophilus bacteria of the bowel, and their high POTASSIUM content benefits the muscular system.

BEETS: Beets are good for the gallbladder and liver. They contain many minerals. They are high in VITAMIN A and are therefore valuable for the eliminative, lymphatic, and digestive systems.

BLACKBERRIES: Blackberries are high in IRON but can cause constipation. They have been used to control diarrhea. If tolerated, blackberry juice is one of the finest builders of the blood.

BLUEBERRIES: Blueberries contain silicon, which rejuvenates the pancreas.

BROCCOLI: Broccoli is best eaten with protein, which helps drive the amino acids to the brain. It is high in VITAMIN A and C and low in calories. It is helpful to the eliminative system.

CABBAGE: This is one of the least expensive of the vitamin-protective foods. It is an excellent source of VITAMIN C. Cooked red cabbage is superior to white or green. The outside leaves have as much as 40 percent more CALCIUM than the inside leaves. It is helpful in overcoming consti-pation. Sauerkraut is good for a sluggish intestinal tract and serious cases of constipation. Cabbage helps to keep a clean, clear complexion.

CARROTS: Carrots are extremely high in VITAMIN A, which helps improve eyesight. They contain much roughage and are helpful in constipation. Carrot juice is a general body builder.

CAULIFLOWER: The greatest amount of CALCIUM in cauliflower is found in the greens that surround the head. They can be cooked with the heads or used in salads. Cauliflower can cause gas.

CELERY: Its high water content makes it a perfect accompani-ment to heavy starches. The greener the stalks, the higher the VITAMIN A. It is rich in CHLORINE, sodium, POTASSIUM, and MAGNESIUM. Celery is best eaten raw. The leaves are rich in POTASSIUM, sodium, and sulfur. The raw leaves are excellent in treating diabetes. They are also helpful to the nerves and for all acid conditions of the body.

CHERRIES: Cherries are high in IRON and therefore an excellent laxative and blood builder. They are also an effective gall-bladder and liver cleanser. Cherries combine well with other fruits and with proteins, but not with starches. They should not often be mixed with dairy foods.

CRANBERRIES: Cranberries have a heavy acid content. They are best if cooked, with raisins and a little honey added to

sweeten. They are useful as a remedy for rectal disturbances, piles, urinary-tract infections, hemorrhoids, and
inflammation.

CUCUMBERS: They are a digestive aid and have a purifying
effect on the bowel. They have a cooling effect on the
blood.

EGGPLANTS: They contain a large amount of water. They are
good for balancing diets that are heavy in protein and
starches.

ENDIVE: Endive is high in VITAMIN A and works very well in
ridding the body of infections. It is high in IRON and
POTASSIUM. It is best eaten raw.

FIGS: Figs are best eaten raw and fresh; however, dried figs
also have nutrients. Figs are a laxative because of the
pectin they contain. They are high in CALCIUM and carbohydrates and turn into energy very quickly. When fresh,
they mix well with all fruits. Dried figs mix well with
starches, vegetables, and subacid fruits. They do not mix
with acidic foods such as TOMATOES and citrus fruits.

GARLIC: Garlic has often been considered a medicinal plant
and a natural antibiotic. It is high in IODINE and sulfur.
Mixed with PARSLEY, it helps high blood pressure.

GRAPEFRUIT: They are rich in VITAMIN C, B_1, and B_2, and low
in calories. They are very rich in POTASSIUM, CALCIUM, citric acids, and salts. The juice can be taken in the evening
to encourage a sound sleep. They are helpful in reducing
fevers from colds and the flu and seldom cause allergic
reactions. They contain vitamin P, which is important for
healthy gums and teeth.

GRAPES: Grapes are considered highly therapeutic due to their
high MAGNESIUM content. Magnesium is needed for regular
bowel movements. Grapes promote the action of the bowel,
cleanse the liver, and aid in kidney function. They are alka-

linizing to the blood and high in water content, so they add
to the fluids necessary to eliminate hardened deposits found
within the body. Dark grapes are high in IRON.

LEEKS: They are suitable for throat disorders and acute nasal
discharges, because they loosen the phlegm. Leeks are a
useful blood purifier and aid in the health of the liver and
the respiratory system.

LEMONS: Lemon juice is an outstanding source of VITAMIN C.
It must be fresh, though. Lemons are high in POTASSIUM
and rich in VITAMIN B$_1$. They are ideal for getting rid of
toxic materials in the body. They are good for throat
trouble and tend to help fevers.

LENTILS: They neutralize muscle acids in the body and are
good for the heart. They mix with vegetables and grains
to provide a rich supply of minerals and protein.

LETTUCE: Leaf lettuce is the reference—head lettuce is virtually empty of nutrients, other than water. Lettuce juice
helps promote sleep. The darker green the leaves, the
higher the vitamin content.

LIMA BEANS: Fresh beans have a high protein value. One
pound of lima beans contains as many nutrients as two
pounds of meat. Dry beans have a higher protein content
than fresh.

MELONS: They give an excellent supply of water that contains
many mineral elements. Melons are considered a rejuve-
nator and alkaline inducer for the body. Melons are also
excellent for aiding elimination.

MUSHROOMS: Mushrooms are among the few rich sources of
germanium, which increases oxygen efficiency of the
body, combatting the effects of pollution. They also contain VITAMIN B.

ONIONS: They contain large amounts of sulfur and are good
for the liver. They mix well with proteins. Parsley helps

neutralize the effects of the onion sulfur in the intestinal tract.

ORANGES: Oranges are excellent sources of VITAMIN C. They are helpful for overacidic body conditions, constipation, or a particularly sluggish intestinal tract. Oranges aid in elimination. They are an excellent source for overall good health.

PAPAYAS: They are rich in vitamins, especially A, C, and E. They are also rich in IRON, PHOSPHORUS, and CALCIUM. Papayas are high in digestive properties and have a direct tonic effect on the stomach and are, therefore, often used in treatment of stomach ulcers.

PARSLEY: It is a blood purifier and a stimulant to the bowel. It is high in IRON and rich in COPPER and MANGANESE. Many kidney complaints will decrease when parsley is added to the diet.

PARSNIPS: Parsnips improve bowel action and have a beneficial effect on the liver. They are slightly diuretic. They are similar to CARROTS in food value.

PEACHES: Peaches are high in VITAMIN A. They also serve as a laxative to the body. They help stimulate digestive juices, are easy to assimilate, and are excellent for children and the elderly. They aid in toxin elimination.

PEARS: Pears are high in VITAMIN C and IRON. They are a digestive aid and help normalize bowel activity.

PEAS: Peas are an excellent source of VITAMIN A, B_1, and C. The pods are very high in chlorophyll, IRON, and CALCIUM-controlling properties. They are slightly diuretic. They also give relief to ulcer pains in the stomach by using up the stomach acids. In the case of ulcers, peas should be puréed.

PEPPERS, GREEN AND RED: They contain many nutrients that resist infections. They contain VITAMIN A, B, and C.

Green peppers are high in silicon, which is needed for healthy hair, skin, nails, and teeth.

PINEAPPLES: They are beneficial for constipation and poor digestion. They help digest proteins.

PLUMS AND PRUNES: Dried prunes are good for the nerves because of their PHOSPHORUS content. Prunes have a laxative effect. Fresh plums are more acidic than fresh prunes. Too many plums may cause an overacidic reaction.

POTATOES: They contain alkaline POTASSIUM, which promotes liver action, elastic tissues, and supple muscles. They seem to help build the left side of the body (which is the heart and intestinal side).

PUMPKINS: They are high in POTASSIUM and sodium. They are a fair source of VITAMIN B and C.

RADISHES: They are strongly diuretic and stimulate the appetite and digestion.

RASPBERRIES: They are considered an effective cleanser for mucus and toxins in the body. They are a good source of VITAMIN A and C.

SPINACH: It is an excellent source of VITAMIN C, VITAMIN A, and IRON and contains about 40 percent POTASSIUM. It promotes the health of the lymphatic, urinary, and digestive systems. Spinach can have a laxative effect and is good for weight-loss diets. The body is unable to utilize the CALCIUM found in cooked spinach.

SQUASH: Winter varieties contain more VITAMIN A than summer varieties. All are high in POTASSIUM and help the elimination system.

STRAWBERRIES: They are high in VITAMIN C. They are fairly high in POTASSIUM and sodium. Hives from strawberries often come from fruit not ripened on the vine. In addition to avoiding "store-ripened" berries, another possible solution is to run hot water over the berries, then cold water. This is believed to remove the fuzz, which may cause hives.

SWEET POTATOES: They are very high in VITAMIN A and niacin.

SWISS CHARD: It is high in VITAMIN C and A, POTASSIUM, sodium, and CALCIUM. Do not overcook. It is helpful to the digestive system.

TOMATOES: Tomatoes increase the alkalinity of the blood and help remove toxins, especially uric acid. They make effective blood and liver cleansers. They are high in vitamins.

Notes

Chapter Two: What Is Wellness?
1. Melvyn R. Werbach, *Nutritional Influences of Illness: A Sourcebook of Clinical Research* (Tarzana, CA: Third Line Press, 1987).

Chapter Seven: Where Do I Start?
1. Marilyn Diamond, *The American Vegetarian Cookbook from the Fit for Life Kitchen* (New York: Warner Books, 1990), page 3.
2. N. M. Walker, *Diet and Salad* (Prescott, AZ; Norwalk Press, 1986), page 24, emphasis added.
3. John A. McDougall, *McDougall's Medicine: A Challenging Second Opinion* (Piscataway, NJ: New Century Publishers, 1985), page 290, emphasis added.
4. Luc De Schepper, *Full of Life* (Los Angeles: Tale Weaver Publishing, 1991), page 22.
5. Dr. John Yudkin, Physician, Biochemist, Emeritus Professor of Nutrition at London University, quoted in Kathy Hishigo, *The Art of Dieting Without Dieting* (Glendale, CA: The Self-Sufficiency Association, 1986).
6. *New York Times*, July 12, 1988, page 1.

7. The aliases for MSG include: Accent, Vetsin, Chinese seasoning, Glutavene, RL-50, hydrolyzed vegetable protein (HVP), hydrolyzed plant protein, natural flavors (may be HVP), or flavorings.

Chapter Eight: Go for the Gold
1. H. Tomlinson, circa 1958, emphasis added.

Appendix A: Cleanses
1. Jason Serius, ed., *Psychoimmunity and the Healing Process: A Holistic Approach to Immunity and AIDS* (Millbrae, CA: Celestial Arts, 1986), pages 211-212.
2. Paul C. and Patricia Bragg, *The Miracle of Fasting* (Santa Barbara, CA: Health Science, 1984), page 22.

Author

Cheryl Townsley is president of Lifestyle for Health, a company committed to helping people learn how to develop healthy lifestyles. Her speaking engagements throughout the country include Fortune 500 companies, women's groups, and general conferences. She has taught cooking classes through health-food stores and public schools since 1989. Cheryl has been featured on several television shows and radio talk shows.

Since 1991 Cheryl has published a national, bimonthly newsletter entitled *Lifestyle for Health Newsletter*. In addition, she has self-published three cookbooks: *Lifestyle for Health*, *Meals in 30 Minutes*, and *Kid's Favorites*. She also distributes tapes, manuals, and booklets promoting practical, healthy living.

Cheryl resides in Denver, Colorado, with her husband, Forest, and their daughter, Anna.